DEDICATION

This book is dedicated to Lo Lo and Toy Boy, to my father for his gift of courageous fortitude, and to Jason for all he has taught me.

"I'm sorry, Mrs. Bronson. I know this is going to be hard on you. But your son is suffering from hepatitis B. We found morphine in his blood. The kid's on the needle. He's an addict. . . ."

The Critics Hail Jill Ireland's
LIFE LINES

"A wrenching and gripping true-life ordeal. . . . Jill Ireland writes with style and compassion."
—Jackie Collins

*   *   *

"A woman of tremendous strength and charm. . . . Excruciating but poignant memories."
—Los Angeles Times

*   *   *

"This autobiography is a manual on how to come to grips with personal tragedy by getting to the bottom of it."
—Newsweek

*   *   *

"A big winner . . . Ireland hits her stride as a writer and presents a fiercely superior book."
—Kirkus Reviews

*   *   *

"Intensely personal. . . . Suffused with pathos and love and pride."
—West Coast Review of Books

*   *   *

"Written with love, understanding, and honesty that offers help to people who have had to confront similar struggles. . . . Jill Ireland has proven she is a fighter . . . in an extraordinarily open, honest, unsparing look at the author as wife, mother, and star."
—Marlboro Enterprise/Hudson Daily Sun (Marlboro, MA)

*   *   *

"Moving and uplifting."
—Dallas Morning News

Also by
JILL IRELAND

LIFE WISH

LIFE LINES

JILL IRELAND

WARNER BOOKS

A Time Warner Company

WARNER BOOKS EDITION

Cover design by Andrew Newman
Cover photo by Roddy McDowall

Warner Books, Inc.
666 Fifth Avenue
New York, N.Y. 10103

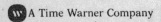 A Time Warner Company

Printed in the United States of America

This book was originally published in hardcover by Warner Books.
First Printed in Paperback: December, 1990

10 9 8 7 6 5 4 3 2 1

ACKNOWLEDGMENTS

I would like to thank William Sarnoff and Nansey Neiman of Warner Books for their initial encouragement and confidence in this book. I send my gratitude to Jamie Raab and Gail Rebuck for their helpful suggestions. Special thanks go to my fine editor, Vernon Scott. To my family, the Bronsons, Irelands, and McCallums, I give my love and abiding appreciation for their forbearance. And to my mother, Dorothy Eborn Ireland, my love for her strength and wisdom.

CHAPTERS

CONTENTS

CONTENTS

LIFE
LINES

A Baby is Lost

Bavaria, Germany

June 1961

I was twenty-five years and six weeks old.

I lay in bed in a sterile little hotel room in Possenhoffen, Germany. I had been in terrible pain for some time. I was alone. My husband, David, was out frantically searching for a doctor as the switchboard of the hotel was unmanned.

After four hours of torment the soft tissues of my body relaxed. For a brief moment I was relieved of pain; my senses had turned inward, making me aware of the innermost secret parts of me in a way I had never experienced before. A primitive urge impelled me to get out of the bed. Weakly, I squatted on the floor. Then, in a sudden, unexpected rush, pain pierced me and tore me apart. Something deep inside my body moved, rushing, falling out of control. A feeling of horror, then warm wet relief as emptiness followed what before had been the compacted pressure of fullness.

A slippery object about the size of a loaf of bread was lying on the floor between my legs. I began to scream. I had miscarried my baby. I saw it would have been my son.

1

A Baby is Born

Los Angeles, California

Kaboom! Kaboom! Kaboom!

The steady, reassuring sound that Kier had heard since he existed was becoming more intense, insistent, while somehow fading into the distance. Kier felt a tragic sadness coupled with excitement as every cell in his being fought to become free, to emerge in his own right, to hear his own voice, see with his own eyes, smell and taste for himself, all that until now Vicky had done for him.

For nine months he had been growing in the warm, nurturing womb. In the last four months he listened, aware of the conflict going on in the space that surrounded the woman who carried him. The sound and feel of sobbing shook him as the body that held him was racked with crying. Loud voices, angry words. He heard confidences addressed to him.

"Oh, my baby, what shall I do?"

Kier heard, understood to the depths of his soul. He was part of the sorrow and yet apart. He was doing what his fate decreed; he was growing, getting stronger, pushing against the confines of the enclosing walls, stretching his curled-up arms and legs. Occasionally he sucked his thumb.

The grief disturbed him. "Don't weep, Mother. I will soon be with you. I will hold you, love you. I will dry your tears."

Kier longed for the day when he would see the face of the woman who already had given him so much of herself.

His mother's heartbeat picked up its rhythm. He thought he heard her cry out as cold steel seized his head. Then he was pulled, protesting, drawing back, shrieking at the ghastly wrench.

His mother's body was loath to give him up.

Now he heard her cry. Her tears mingling with his own. He was surrounded by white light, his body wrapped in a strange foreign substance. Never again would he feel the smooth slick warmth in which he had lived those last intimate months. The sense of loss was intolerable.

Then she was there, holding him. He knew it. He made out a cloud of dark hair and dark eyes in a face with skin as smooth and white as the light around him. Then he knew it had all been worthwhile. Now they were truly together.

He felt her insert her finger into his hand. He made a fist, holding on tightly.

Mother. He knew the word. He had heard it while he was growing inside her. This is my mother.

She lifted him close to her face. He felt her breath, smelled her skin, her warmth. She gave him her breast and guided her firm, elongated nipple between his lips. He grasped it, sucking hungrily. Hot colostrum began to flow into his mouth.

My mother.

The intensity of his fierce love burned his soul as he suckled. She kissed him, then tightened her arms about him and said, "I love you, my son, my baby."

It was a moment held in time.

They took him away, wrapped in his new blanket. They gave him a bottle with a rubber nipple to replace his mother's warm, soft body. He roared; he flailed his fists in anger. He fought. He called her as he was placed on his back in a small white bed. Now he was tired. The milk warmed him. Then, in spite of his grief, he fell asleep.

While he slept, his mother signed the papers and quietly left the hospital.

Each day they came for him, fed, bathed, and clothed him. He cried because they were not his mother. Then one day they told him he was being prepared to be taken to her. His heart sang. He lay quietly, contentedly, while they took care of him. Soon he would be back in her arms, close to the heart that beat with the same intense emotional energy of his own.

It had been two days since they had been separated and his body craved the physical chemistry of her, magical changes that would take place when their flesh touched.

Kier had been so lonely in his clean little hospital crib. He needed his mother. The aroma, touch, and taste of her. He missed the sound of her voice with its soft burr. It would be clear now that her body would not be muffling the sound. Soon they would be one again. Soon.

Mother. Oh, Mother. He was full of longing.

They were taking him to her now, carrying him down a long, dimly lit corridor, down. Down, down, down. It took a long time. Then they burst into a room full of daylight.

"Here he is," someone said. "Your baby."

And they placed him in his mother's arms. They were warm, soft arms, but they smelled different. He relaxed his body and tried to reestablish the bond he knew so well, but the heartbeat of the mother who held him was quicker and lighter. He could not blend with it. They were somehow out of synchronization.

He turned his head to the soft breast, searched with his mouth for the place that had nurtured him. Small nostrils flared, seeking the smell of her, but he could not find it. The yearning grew worse. His body was on edge, poised for the release that the chemistry between them would deliver. He needed that warm, swooning sensation, but it did not come.

In dismay, he looked up into the light, his body screaming for relief, his eyes searching for the dark ones so like his own, for the cloud of black hair. His heartbeat skipped as he saw the halo of gold around her face and bright blue eyes.

It wasn't her! It was not his mother. He began to wail, primitively, sadly keening, knowing he had lost her.

Then he felt the golden-haired one begin to rock him in her arms, fill him with her energy. It was the same primitive maternal love of two days earlier, but it was more a crystal stream of love that would flow into a surging river, then down into an endless ocean, a strong current of love.

She spoke in a quiet voice meant just for him. He stopped crying.

"Hello," she said. "Hello there, Jason. I love you, little boy. I'll take care of you."

Kier lay still in her arms. She gently removed the blanket from his face and opened it.

"He's so beautiful," she said. "Look, such lovely dark eyes and all that curly dark hair. Oh, my."

She held him closer. "He's beautiful."

The man beside her spoke. "We better be going; get him home."

A dark head bent over him. A large, hard but gentle hand touched his head.

"Hello, you," the man said. "Well, come on, Jill; we'll take Jason home."

Then, although his heart and soul cried out for his mother and his body craved her, Kier was carefully carried by this kind but foreign stranger out of the place of his birth and into the world.

He would never see his mother again. It was over. His body would have to learn new rhythms, a new language of love.

He would have to adjust, to fit in to this other energy that surrounded him, a very different energy from the one of which he was forged, more subtle and insistent. But it was strong. He felt the power as he lay cradled in her arms. He felt the love growing stronger each moment. He knew he could live with his new love, but would he survive without her? He would have to change, to become someone else. No longer was it enough just to exist, a part of a whole. Now he had to be what she expected, this new mother called Jill.

She doesn't know me. She will discover me day by day. She will explore my soul. She will know nothing about me through inherited instinct. We will have to learn about each other. Nothing will be chemical. No inherited knowledge. She's warm and safe. She loves me.

I'm not at home in her arms. I'm not happy. I am lonely. Perhaps it will get better. But where is Mother? Is she all right? I'll never know now.

He began to cry again.

Good-bye, Mother. I love you. I always will.

Exhausted, Kier fell asleep on the bottle that his new mother put in his mouth.

2

Shepherd's Bush

December 1909

My father was born in 1905 to Florence and Frederick Ireland in the Shepherd's Bush district of London, where they lived in a narrow, pungent, straw and manure-strewn mews close to a green commons. Frederick was a coachman and hostler who worked hard and long to support his family. Jack was his seventh child. His siblings were Fred, Harold, Albert, Annie, Elsie (his favorite), and Louisa. Younger than Jack was Ellen, who died very young, as did Annie.

Jack awoke each morning to the sound of the heavy hooves of carriage horses on the stone streets, which excited and aroused him. Peeping out of the window he would squint while peering through the mist, listening to the clopping. In the early dawn light the men, until his eyes accustomed themselves to the gloom, appeared as gray ghosts in the ever-present London fog. The hostlers were, for the most part, gaunt and pale. They stamped their feet and blew onto cold hands. Scarves over their mouths kept out the grime and chill. Jack pressed his face to the window to see the line of cabbies moving along the mews in the biting cold, steam rising from newly deposited piles of horse droppings. Brave banter raised their spirits and breath from their lungs condensed and mingled in the air. From where he sat, Jack was entranced by the masculine world outside, the men with their jokes and their power over the large, lumbering beasts. This was life to Jack, a man's world he could not wait to join. Jack loved horses, their smell, the soft muzzles. He wanted to grow up quickly, to become part of life in the stables.

Frederick taught him to care for the animals, how to whistle before putting them away in their stalls. He told the amazed little boy this caused the horses to relieve themselves of vast quantities of streaming water, thereby saving their bedding from becoming sodden.

Unlike some cabbies, Frederick cared for the animal he drove each day. He had a relationship with the horse. He brought small tidbits from his table, stale bread or an apple core left over after he himself had eaten the fruit. He showed his son how to blow gently into the horse's nostrils and then turn his head so the animal could return the communication by nuzzling and blowing warm air in the little boy's hair.

"Take your hat off, Jack," Frederick would tell him. "Let him smell your hair. Let him smell your head. That way he will always know you."

The love of horses was the strongest, most lasting part of himself that Frederick left John Alfred Ireland, my father, and he also passed on to his son an inherited fortitude that would stand little Jack in good stead. That and one final happy memory.

It began early on a special morning when Frederick Ireland took Jack along on his rounds. Jack sat beside his father, bundled up against the cold in a coat belonging to an older brother and a cloth cap pulled down over his ears against the chill. Condensed moisture rose from his breath as the child in a piping voice encouraged the large, dark-brown cart horse to "Walk on, Boy."

Surreptitiously, his father tapped the old horse on its

flanks and winked at his friend, a fellow hostler. "See you later, Herb," Frederick said. "It'll be an easy day for me with my mate here to help." Then to Jack he added, "Okay, old son," and placed the reins in the child's fingers while keeping a cautious length of the leather straps in his own hand.

Jack sat proudly, never minding the biting cold. His father coughed hackingly and spat into the street. Jack copied him, spitting manfully. Breathing this morning was a painful endeavor for Frederick. The tightness and burning in his chest had worsened. Although still a young man by twentieth-century standards, Frederick suffered chronic fatigue; lassitude was ever present. It took great concentration to simply breathe. He sat in the cold anticipating the many hours of discomfort that stretched out ahead of him. Having the bright-eyed, eager little boy with him gave Frederick animal comfort. He pulled the child closer to him as one would a warm puppy, and started down the mews.

Frederick looked up as was his custom to see his wife, Florence. Her round, smooth, sloe-eyed face smiled back from the window. She waved to them as they moved out of sight. Their day had begun.

Fred Ireland watched the boy as he competently drove the carriage. He was proud of Jack, his youngest son. He thought of Flo and how, when they first met, his friends had chanted an old London rhyme, "Change the name and not the letter. Change for worse and not for better."

"Ha! So much for that," he muttered to himself.

Frederick Ireland was most happy with this Florence Isles. This was one instance, he congratulated himself, that blending the letters *I*—Ireland and Isles—had worked out very well. And look at the fine young son their passion had begot.

Frederick pulled his topcoat more closely around his throat. He felt the chill and missed the muffler that he had wound around his child's neck. He leaned back behind the open seat and lifted out the old, soiled, much-used horse blanket and put it around himself.

"Sorry, mate," he said to the horse, "I need it more than you today."

It would be a long cold day for the cabbie.

To keep their spirits up Frederick began to sing a song that Jack would one day teach his own children and grand-children:

Horsey, keep your tail up,
Keep your tail up,
Keep your tail up,
And keep the sun out of my eyes.
Tell me how you get that way.
I say yes, but you say neigh, neigh.
Horsey, keep your tail up and keep the sun out of my eyes.

Neither father nor son was daunted by the inappropri-ateness of the weather described in the song. The sun would not shine that day, nor would it shine much longer in the life of Frederick Ireland.

Later that night Florence heard the two of them caroling "Show me the way to go home" as the old horse kerlip-kerlopped through the mews in the December night. Flor-ence shook her head with resignation. She knew their clothes would be soaked through to the skin as they sat high and exposed on the hard wooden seat. It had begun to sleet.

It was this night that caused Frederick's bronchitis to worsen and develop into pneumonia. The next day he was forced to his bed. He would never guide the old horse and cab back home again.

3

Los Angeles, California

January 14, 1962

The day the baby was born, my husband was in Arizona. The next day, my lover was with me at the small private clinic in downtown Los Angeles where I was to pick up my new infant son.

A redheaded nurse brought the baby to me. She held the bundle possessively as if she did not want to part with it. She looked at me almost suspiciously, as if sizing up my ability to take on this responsibility. Finally, she placed the baby in my arms, saying, "Take good care of him."

"I will," I said, holding the warm little body close to me. My lover and I parted the blanket to peer at the baby's face. He looked at us in a puzzled way. He had a shock of dark hair and a rather mature face for such a newborn. Together we drove him back to the house in which I was living with Paul, my four-year-old son.

On the way, I asked Charles, "Do you think he feels funny being driven in the car?"

He responded, "All the bumping and swaying probably makes him feel he's still in the womb."

So, it was in a big black Cadillac convertible with its black leather interior that the infant made his debut out into the world, leaving behind him the dark-haired twenty-six-year-old girl whom I knew to be the same age as myself. She believed she was giving her son a chance at a better life than the one she could provide. With great generosity of spirit, she had blessed the child and prayed for his happy future.

I was the proud mother of a beautiful, two-day-old infant. The bonding was immediate and for life. My husband agreed we would name him Jason David McCallum.

At home I quickly discovered Jason was a troubled little baby.

From the very beginning there was always a different energy emanating from him, one as unlike mine as chalk to cheese. His energy blew with an almost Eastern heat and sensuality, an energy that demanded instant gratification and satisfaction. He needed all my attention, something I gave with pleasure and love.

I no sooner fed him and laid him down in a small basket crib than he emitted a loud, demanding roar, which crumpled his face, turning it puce. He wrinkled his dark-haired, furry skull while his small wiry body went into a spasmodic, tight-fisted fury. These Olympian efforts sometimes caused his crib to career on its wheeled legs across the linoleum floor of the kitchen where I had placed it to watch him as I cooked a small meal for Paul and myself.

The first few days with Jason were all sorting out, getting to know him, his rhythms, his personality, which at only two days of age was a determined one. He cried for hours. He dropped weight. He was a most unhappy infant.

He appeared to be in a great deal of pain. His small body trembled as his arms and legs stretched out, his fingers grasping into the air around him as if trying to catch onto something, reaching as if for a lifeline. I did my best to comfort him. I carried him for hours, patting his back soothingly, then gently jiggling him up and down in the age-old way that women instinctively know.

He had thrush, an uncomfortable mouth fungus, contracted in his natural mother's birth canal. He had a sensitive digestive system. He was unable to keep milk down.

It was always the same. He would finish the last drop, cradled cozily in my arms, then with an explosive burst of energy the whole bottle would come back up, gushing fountains of sour milk that never failed to soak my clothing and often my hair.

The baby had trouble sleeping. I spent nights cuddling and walking him to relieve the grippe spasms. His little face and body would contract painfully. His screams were impressive.

He had dreadful gas bubbles, his dark face contorted with the effort to relieve them. He was beset with miseries, awake all the time, crying between feedings, then falling asleep on the bottle.

Jason was allergic to cows' milk and evaporated milk. All kinds of milk. He was in an uproar, devastated by the denial of mother's milk, that basic necessity I was unable to supply.

I considered buying a nanny goat, but finally the child accepted a brand of powdered milk and for a while we both got some sleep.

When Jason was two weeks old I wrapped him in a blue hand-knit blanket and took him to our family pediatrician Dr. Arthur Grossman. I was overcome with apprehension. He was going to perform a circumcision.

"Did you bring a bottle, Jill?" the doctor asked.

"Yes, I did."

"Okay, then, this shouldn't take too long. Give me the bottle and wait outside."

He took my precious baby and disappeared into a cubicle with his nurse. My hands were clammy. My heart pounded. My God, I didn't know if they would give him an anesthetic. My poor son. I paced the hallway that ran down the middle of six separate cubicles used for examining little patients. A scream, which I recognized as Jason's, pierced the clinic.

I fainted and knew nothing more until I came round, stretched out on the narrow leather couch in the doctor's office. I opened my eyes and sat up.

Jason was lying on his back in his diapers atop the doctor's desk, happily sucking his bottle.

Dr. Grossman picked him up, came round, and asked, "Are you feeling better, Jill?"

He put my baby in my arms. I searched the infant's face for signs of tears or pain. I kissed the top of his head. Jason, oblivious to my affections, sucked on the nipple like a starveling.

"It was no trouble at all," said the doctor. "He only cried when we took the bottle out of his mouth."

I looked up, incredulous. "Do you mean that's what the awful scream was about?"

The nurse had come into the room and heard my question.

"Uh-huh," she said. "That's what it was all about. He didn't feel the other at all."

But Jason's scream was the beginning of a long and continued identification with his pain, a symbiosis that would exist for many years to come.

Paul loved his little brother and helped me as much as a four-year-old was able. He had wanted a brother very much.

Paul had been aware of my miscarriage and was as disappointed as I about losing a new baby brother or sister. He had repeatedly asked when I would have another baby. I told him the doctors didn't think I could ever bring another child into the world. I discussed with him my decision to adopt.

My son was thrilled with the idea, so one sunny Thursday in August 1961, I took Paul with me on the initial interview at a private adoption agency. I had called ahead to say I wanted to discuss adopting a child. The woman who received us ushered mother and son into an office where we sat in two big wingback chairs facing a large, leather-topped antique desk.

The woman asked if Paul would prefer to sit in an outer office with some crayons.

I said, "Oh, no. This meeting concerns Paul. He knows all about it. And naturally, although he's young, I want him here."

The woman drew back. The proper little English boy's presence seemed to inhibit her. She shuffled some papers on her desk, then looking at me, she said point blank, "Are you sure you want the child to listen to the details of his adoption?"

There had been some confusion. I soon cleared up the misunderstanding.

I was told there was a woman about my age, of Irish descent. The circumstances of her life had left her separated from her husband, living alone with her two young sons. During this period of separation she had developed a relationship with a man of Italian ancestry and conceived. The father, an architect, was married with two sons of his own. Marriage was out of the question.

Recent developments made it appear as if a reconciliation with her husband was possible in the future. However, she knew this would not happen if her estranged spouse discovered she was pregnant by another man. The young woman, refusing to consider abortion, decided to give the baby up for adoption.

My husband, David, still away on a film location, called me the evening after the interview at the agency to get a full report of what had taken place. We agreed to support the natural mother financially through her delivery. The payments were arranged through a lawyer. In exchange for prenatal care, doctor and hospital bills, we agreed to assume custody of the unborn child no matter what problems or handicaps it may have brought into the world. Like natural parents, we were taking our chances.

Because David was busy on the film most of the time, Paul and I spent the first few weeks of Jason's life as a small family unit of three. We were happy and snug. Paul and I loved the baby in spite of his being a twenty-four-hour-a-day job. To me, Jason was the baby I had lost in miscarriage and a further commitment to my marriage.

I've made some hard decisions in my life. I've tried never to look back, never have regrets. Remorse is alien to me. All the same, I do not always sleep the quiet sleep of the blameless.

When I submitted the adoption papers, I fully intended to stay with my marriage. We were a family, David, me, Paul, and Jason. But I was vulnerable and unhappy after my miscarriage. I had nearly died. This love affair was a celebration, giving in to the power and the passion of life. When it began, seven months before the adoption, we both thought it would be just a beautiful moment, something to remember. We didn't mean it to change our lives irrevocably.

The doctors told me I would never bear another child. After the adoption and when David completed the film, we planned to leave the country immediately. Our lives were in England; the months in America unreal. Just a magic moment in time.

I thought the control was all in my hands. But my lover was not a man to be trifled with. I had no idea the film would still be in production when David and I took custody of Jason.

Then when Jason was a mere three months old, after a visit to the Arizona location, I discovered I was pregnant again. I visited a gynecologist who would be my doctor for the next twenty-six years.

Dr. Alexander Culiner was a tall, robust man who had spent a great deal of time practicing in Africa. He was down-to-earth with a no-nonsense personality. He was reassuring and kind. I liked him immediately.

He said, "Try not to be frightened. A pregnancy is like fruit on a tree. If it's going to be good it will stay on the tree, if not, it will drop off."

The doctor watched me as, wide-eyed with fear, I told him of the loss of my baby a mere seven months earlier, and that I was told I could not become pregnant again. I recounted how I hemorrhaged, unable to leave my bed in the hospital for weeks. I could not afford to have that happen again. I had two children to take care of now. I had no family in America to help. I could not afford to be ill. The terrible memories were still fresh. I was terrified it would happen again.

Dr. Culiner placated me. "Be patient. It's quite possible this pregnancy will be perfectly all right. It's happened many times before. A woman can't conceive, or if she does, she can't carry a child to fruition, then she adopts a baby and suddenly finds herself pregnant and has an uncomplicated birth."

Dr. Culiner proved to be right. His quiet confidence convinced me. I settled down into an uncomplicated pregnancy.

I continued caring for Jason, marveling at how handsome he was becoming. He had lustrous dark hair and large, very dark blue eyes, a tiny cleft in his chin. I would lie him outdoors naked and kicking in a large English pram, then watch delightedly as he turned a beautiful golden brown. I felt great maternal pride when people looked beneath the fringed canopy to exclaim what a beautiful baby he was.

My third son lay curled up inside me, listening and waiting, absorbing my emotions and joys, knowing the love I was experiencing, hearing us, as Jason had done in his mother's womb.

When Jason was nine months old I gave birth to a son. David and I named him Valentine Luke. Valentine, a perfect complement to Jason's dark good looks, was flaxen with periwinkle-blue eyes that gleamed with a knowing intelligence. Weighing in at ten pounds, eight ounces, with a length of twenty-two inches, Valentine inspired Dr. Culiner's observation: "This one's been here before."

And, so it seemed, he had. Valentine was ahead in everything. Lying in his crib as a small infant he tried to talk. By this time my lover Charles was a familiar visitor. He found Valentine a fascinating baby. He would lean over the crib and say, "Hello, Valentine, how are you?"

Valentine would watch Charlie's face intently. Then when Charles finished speaking, Valentine would respond.

"Da wabba, ba-boom, ba-boo, ba-boom," involving a lot of action from his tongue, which would flicker in and out of his little mouth as he made his first attempts to speak. He was then scarcely more than two months old. It was clear we would be hearing a lot more from my youngest son.

Meanwhile, Jason crawled around the house, pulling himself up on furniture, generally exploring the world.

The three boys and I were a unit. But Jason was different. Paul and Val came from David and me, two thousand years of English tradition, custom, and that unique gene pool provided by an island people whose character, values, and mores were honed through countless generations of homogenous breeding and tradition. For better or worse, we were alike.

I had memories of my own childhood. I reacted instinctively the way my mother and father did. Eons of DNA connected me to my past, strains of Anglo-Saxon heritage, just as an eternity of DNA connected Jason to his Latin-Celtic background. How different his life would have been had I not plundered his cradle. If he could have known the natural progression of generational evolution of those ancient ancestors, he would have enjoyed shortcuts to the minds and hearts of his natural parents, their intellect and humor. They would have known what to guard him against, flesh of their flesh, aware of their own strengths and weaknesses, forgiven him his, then taken pride in seeing themselves re-created, recognizing Uncle Angelo's business acumen coming to life three generations later, appreciating Uncle Sean's lyrical turn of phrase.

Jason, like a space traveler suspended from the mother ship, had been connected by a lifeline to his birthright and heritage. We cut that line, his mother and I. I came to him an alien and all the love I gave him could never compensate his loss. But back then I was happy and unknowing. I had my baby. Valentine arrived in our midst and Jason had a younger brother. Now Jason was the middle child, a notoriously difficult position.

Jason observed his siblings and for the first year of his life seemed to think it perfectly natural that he had a blond mother, fair father, and two fair brothers. Visitors, however, found the two younger boys an intriguing study in contrasts.

I looked away from the fact that Jason was so different from my natural children (while rejoicing in the difference). I determined Jason would be as much my son as his brothers.

I bludgeoned Jason with set phrases used over and over again, "I love you, my little adopted boy." This, I decided, would accustom him to the sound of the word *adopted* so that he would never find it ugly or shocking. I told him repeatedly how much I loved him and used the term *my boys*, referring to them collectively as if they were all one.

With the full blast of my personality I proceeded to try to blend them all together in my eyes, their eyes, and the eyes of the world. I was unaware that deep inside Jason himself a small figure was drowning in the quicksand of my good intentions. The specter of Kier lived on. But I would not know this for another quarter century.

Blithely, I brushed off inquiries about how different Jason was from the others with the phrase, "that's because he's adopted" as if it were of no importance, when all the time it was of *vital* importance. My blood ran hot, burning with the need to absorb this child with maternal pride into the world as I knew it.

But my world was changing quickly. David and I, sadly, were feeling strain in our marriage. I was in love with Charles Bronson, *Charlie*, which caused me great anguish as I still loved David dearly. David was my family, the father of my children. But at age twenty-six, I could not ignore the claim that Charles had on my feelings. Pain was inevitable. It was only a matter of time and tears before my marriage came to a sorrowful end.

Time would eventually sort all this out, but until it did I spent many years wishing that women could have two husbands. I loved them individually and was never happier than when I was with them both.

Now, when I look back, it seems incredible that although Charlie and I met in 1961, we weren't married until seven years later, October 4, 1968.

4
Kier Rebels

1962

After struggling for two months in dis-ease, craving the unattainable, Kier finally slept. Lulled by the crooning of the new mother and the atmosphere of harmonious warmth that she created, Kier let down his guard and crawled to rest in the dark recesses of the child they called Jason. While he did, Jason flourished. He enjoyed being the center of attention. He liked his brothers' company. He was loved, admired, and he knew it. Then, at the age of eleven months, Kier awoke like a tooth bursting through a tender pink gum. He made his presence known.

Kier had rested a long time. He awakened with terrible, frustrated, lonely anger; deprivation accompanied his every hour. It could be contained no longer.

Jason was playing at a small wooden table with colored pegs. He held a wooden hammer, attempting to knock pegs down through holes bored in the toy bench. He was watched over by Jean, the children's English nanny.

Jason and Jean got along well. The way he looked up at her with huge, black-lashed eyes, she found winning. Jean was affectionate with him and Jason was happy. She encouraged him this day, saying, "That's right. Bang the pegs in. Bang them, Jason."

With cries of "Baa, baa, baa," the little boy haphazardly rained blows on the wooden toy.

Jean was summoned by a small cry from the nursery. She left for the adjoining room where two-month-old baby Valentine had been sleeping. Jason looked around. He did not like being left alone. His mother was downstairs. He called loudly for her, "Mama, Mama, Mama."

Large tears rolled down his cheeks. "Ma! Ma! Ma!" he called through his sobs.

His mother was out of earshot. She did not come up the stairs to him. Jean heard him though. She popped her head into the room.

"Now, be a good boy, Jason. I'll be right back. I just have to change Valentine. He's awake now. You just play with your pegs. There's a good boy."

Gasping with deep, shuddering gulps, Jason watched her leave and closed the door firmly behind her. He felt a fluttering deep in his tummy. An empty, scary feeling filled him, like smoke whirling around. He began to scream.

"I won't be long," called Jean through the closed door.

Kier's rage burst forth, consuming Jason. The fear disappeared. Kier crawled, carrying the wooden hammer, to the big French windows. He looked and saw Jason's reflection in the glass. He struck.

Bang! Bang! Bang! The hammer hit the pane. Then crash!

It was beautiful. Kier was filled with wild joy as the shining, transparent wall shattered the image, and he, Kier, had done it.

Exalted, he laughed as the glass tumbled down around him. Great shards of glittering splinters. He laughed and laughed, intoxicated by the feeling of power.

"Baa, baa, baa!" he shouted. "Baa, baa, baa!"

Jean rushed into the room holding Valentine, her eyes

round with horror. "Oh my God, Jason, you bad boy. What did you do?"

His mother came running, having heard the crash downstairs. She saw her son, naked but for his diaper, sitting amid the broken glass. Crossing the room in three strides, she scooped him up.

"Ma, Ma, Ma," he said, eyes shining, smiling at her as he waved his hammer. Kier was full of importance. "Mama."

Carefully, she picked her way back across the glass-strewn carpet.

"Bang, bang, bang," said Kier. He could feel his mother shaking in shock. But he also felt her controlling herself.

"Yes, darling. Bang, bang. But that was a no-no, Jason. Hurt. Hurt. You could have hurt yourself."

She carried him into the bedroom and tenderly inspected his body, between his toes and through his hair where she found small, sparkling particles of glass. She prized his fingers from the hammer and took it from him, saying, "Jason, you must never do that again. It's hot. Ouch! Hurt! Never do that again."

Then she wrapped him in her cashmere shawl and hugged him tightly, kissing him, burying her face in his warm neck.

"I love you, boy-boy. I love you so much. But don't frighten Mama like that ever again."

The child relaxed in her arms, catching a strand of her long hair in his hand and twisting it around his fingers. She crooned to him, singing softly to the tune of "Bye, Baby Bunting, Daddy's Gone A-Hunting," "Mama loves Jason. Mama loves Jason."

The soft fabric of the cashmere against his skin, the rhythmic rocking of the mother's voice, were a wondrous soporific. His eyes glazed over and he fell asleep. As he did, Kier smiled, satisfied. He withdrew to his dark sleeping place. All was well.

5

Mr. Elms Comes Calling

London 1909

Jack was four when his father, Frederick, died in sad circumstances.

He was, of course, too young to comprehend the meaning of death or the dreadful consequences his father's passing would have on his mother Florence, his sisters, his brothers, and on himself.

Frederick and Florence were patients in the same hospital. Frederick was dying of consumption. Florence was a victim of rheumatoid arthritis, which crippled her legs.

She was desperately worried about her children, temporarily in the care of a neighbor. Would the authorities come nosing about to investigate the welfare of her brood?

Full of blind faith that their doctors would make them well, Florence waited for the day when she and Frederick would be allowed to go home.

Then tragedy.

One drab morning Florence was in her hospital bed, alone and in great pain, when a doctor informed her that her husband had died during the night in the nearby ward, leaving her alone to rear their six children, all under the age of fifteen. It was a numbing blow, but there was scarcely time for mourning and certainly not a moment for self-pity. Florence discharged herself from the hospital that day, making her way with difficulty into the street on metal braces and crutches to see to the funeral arrangements and to look after her children.

Florence struggled gallantly, supporting her family by taking in sewing. Her legs had become so useless they could no longer operate the treadle of the sewing machine, which had been converted to operate by hand. Jack and his sisters often turned the hand crank while Florence stitched. The children helped their mother remake an old skirt, patch a cloak, or mend a jacket that would fetch about sixpence and take most of the day to do. Many customers did not pay up and the children, who delivered the work, were told to make sure they had the money in hand before they left the garments.

Life was harsh and worrisome for Florence. But determinedly she kept her family together even under pressure to put the youngest ones in an orphanage.

Jack never forgot his terror as a child at the specter of becoming a public ward. Once a week the youngest children huddled together on the the staircase peeping through the banister rails as their mother, leaning heavily on her crutches, answered the door.

This caller was a kindly man, Jack supposed, but as a boy of six and seven he shivered with fear at the sight of him. Jack dreaded the day Mr. Ernest Elms came calling. He feared the prospect of being led away, never to set eyes on his mother or siblings again.

Jack was haunted by the man's deep basso saying, "Can we take a couple of them, Mrs. Ireland, to help you out?"

On occasion Mr. Elms would glance up at the white, frightened faces of the Ireland children as he spoke.

One night Jack, his breathing shallow with nerves, sat in

his worn gray nightshirt, hugging scrawny knees, his elbows and feet chafed and rough from the cold, chilblains tingling his fingers. His nose was running, his fingernails were dirty, and his bony, little boy's rump found little comfort on the cold, uncarpeted wooden staircase. Beside him sat his sister Elsie, her large brown eyes wide with apprehension. The children drew back in the shadows as the door was opened, not wanting to attract attention to themselves.

"How 'bout those two little 'uns?" said Mr. Elms one unforgettable night, looking meaningfully at Jack and Elsie. The two drew close together and held their breaths until they heard their mother answer firmly, "No. It's all right. I can manage a little longer."

And manage she did while even the youngest of Florence's offspring scrambled to bring home a copper or two to keep the family going.

6

The Boys

1960s

Tanned by the California sunshine, my boys grew rapidly. They played on the terrace behind the Hollywood Hills house. Jason toddled around followed by Val in a walker with wheels. Jason and Val were always together. The two names became linked, almost like twins'.

Valentine shared Jason's room from birth. To forestall sibling rivalry, I had told Jason that Valentine was *his* baby until he began taking that too literally. Jason would climb into his brother's crib and undress him. When that was accomplished he would polish the wall behind the crib with Valentine's diapers. I decided perhaps this wasn't a good idea so I bought Jason a life-size baby doll, saying *this* was Jason's baby, hoping he would exercise his paternal feelings on the doll, which he did in many ways. But every morning when I entered the boys' room I found Jason asleep beside Valentine. I tried to get into the room before they awoke, but Jason had always climbed out of his crib and into Val's to cuddle up to his brother.

I enjoyed my boys enormously. They were all so different. Paul had a loving, trusting intellect. Being my firstborn, he was very special to me. He helped with the younger boys, the more so after David and I separated.

Paul was my number-one son and loving protector. He and I had traveled far together from our English roots. To help fill the void when David left, I bought a half German shepherd half coyote I named Daisy. Then Paul was given a huge bassett hound we called Gregory. A black Persian cat named Henry completed our family.

The Hillside Avenue house sat high on a quiet, tree-lined street established in the California stucco era of the 1930s when homes were commonly painted pastel yellows, greens, blues, and pinks. This one was white with a red-tiled Spanish roof. Three levels faced the plains of Los Angeles with a sweeping vista of the basin and two floors looked out on the Hollywood Hills wilderness of chapparal, sandalwood, yucca, and sage wherein dwelt coyotes, rattlesnakes, raccoons, and other varmints, even the occasional deer.

The house had three bedrooms, but what I loved most was its welcoming personality. On opening the carved black wood door—complete with peephole behind a wrought-iron grille—one stepped into a red-tiled entryway opening onto the dining room on the left and the living room on the right with its deep fireplace and large, arched stained-glass window. On the far side of the room, two steps up led to an alcove in which stood my easel and painting paraphernalia. The shelves in this nook held my books and music.

The ceilings throughout were heavy old wooden beams. I always loved coming through the front door to call: "Boys!" and know they would hear me immediately. Often I could see them playing the moment I came in.

The dining-room arches held a birdcage with a yellow canary called Tweety Pie. He was accustomed to flying merrily around the dining room before landing at one end of the polished dining table and sliding the length of this runway on his fluffy yellow belly, his landing gear tucked up out of sight to avoid skid marks.

David and I bought the house together in 1963, having tendered a modest down payment. When we separated, I took over the payments. I loved the house and decided to hang on to it.

I commonly put Jason on my left hip, his brown legs and arms wrapped tightly around me, and picked up Val with my right arm and sat him on the other hip. I would dash down two flights of stairs from my front door to the garage, with Paul, Daisy, and Gregory bringing up the rear. I was young and strong in those days. David, in the first flush of success of the television series "The Man from U.N.C.L.E.," had bought himself a Corvette Stingray sports car. He telephoned from Italy to ask if I would like to take over the payments. Since I was working in a TV series, I was able to do so.

The sleek, pale-blue Stingray convertible was perfect for me. I managed to jam Paul, Jason, and Val into the single seater while Daisy crawled into the confined space behind it. Gregory remained at home to bay at intruders. Then off we'd go, top down, singing loudly as the air blew our hair around in the sunshine. We all loved the feeling of abandoned freedom.

It was in this car that five-year-old Jason, munching on a cookie and possessively holding on to me with one small arm, asked, "Mudder, when I go in the Army will you pick me up?"

I remember sadness and fright that he might be wounded in a war. If I had known then what real threats were in store for Jason, would I have done anything differently? Did I spoil him? Overcompensate for his being my only adopted child?

Unconditional love is something I thought every child should receive as a birthright. I gave this to Jason. It was easy. He was a funny, sweet little boy, but he always had a different energy from my other children. Even I had to admit that at times he was stubborn and willful.

Jason loved to do little jobs for me. When he was three he designated himself captain of the wastebaskets. He would empty them and reline the baskets with plastic bags. He was happy with his job, proud to be a garbage man. He even had his own supply of dark-green trash bags.

At three he made friends with the gardener. Every day at ten o'clock Jason went to the freezer, removed two Popsicles, one for him and one for James. Together, companionably chatting, they could be seen sitting on the curb in front of the house enjoying their break.

Jason loved soft fabrics; his tactile senses were most important to him. "Henry, oh, Henry," he would say as he gently stroked the cat's soft black fur.

I dreaded facing the confrontational day when I must tell him he was not born of my flesh. So he heard the word *adopted* applied so often that he misunderstood. Jason thought I was saying *doctor*, and he used to practice on Valentine.

When Jason was three and Valentine two, I began working in the TV series "Shane." Weekdays I arose at five o'clock in the morning.

It was a delight on Saturdays to awaken in my four-poster bed to the sound of my little boy singing in the back garden while picking flowers for his mama. Jason would put them in a small vase and bring them to me when Helia, the Mexican housekeeper, brought me my morning tea.

At three Jason's love for Charlie had developed into a passionate obsession that expressed itself suddenly one day while Charlie, Valentine, Jason, and I were all at lunch. Jason, kneeling in the red-leather booth between Charlie and me, suddenly stood up on the seat, grabbed Charlie by the throat and kissed him passionately on the mouth. Charlie was dumbfounded, as were we all.

His was a loving, compassionate nature flowing from a

uniquely attractive face and a small, wiry body, coupled with boundless energy and a zany sense of humor. He loved above all things to laugh. Oh, yes, fun was very important to Jason, more than knowledge, eating, or sleeping. Nothing came easily to him, including nursery school, which he eagerly anticipated. His first few weeks were full of tales about the problems he was having with a character named Red Carney.

Then his stories changed, becoming more romantic. Jason was in love and it was, "My girlfriend this . . . My girlfriend that . . . My girlfriend says . . ."

One day he came home in a black mood, dragging his coat. He threw down his lunchpail with a clatter. Red Carney had stolen his girlfriend.

"But, Jason," we asked, "how can that be? What happened?"

I was indignant. How dare this Red Carney person steal my son's girlfriend?

Jason looked at me with a philosophical, man-of-the-world, pained expression. He shrugged his shoulders, held up his small hands, and said, "I didn't have enough money."

We never learned another thing about Red or the girl-friend. We never mentioned either of them again, but it was obviously a lesson well learned.

The boys and I went to Paris to visit Charlie, who was working in a film. Jason took a great liking to our chauffeur, Blackjack. Jason would sit on the armrest in the front seat of the limousine and place his hands on the man's shoulders. I would see him pat the driver gently. It seemed as if he were always trying to find someone special for himself, just for him; men and women alike.

Blackjack was flattered. One evening he took Jason to his home for the night. Charlie and I were a little concerned. It was a first for Jason. At three in the morning there was a knock on the door. It was a weary French driver holding Jason by the hand.

"He had a good time," Blackjack said, "playing with my sons. But he couldn't seem to settle down when it was time for bed. My wife made him hot chocolate and gave him cookies, but I think he wants his mother."

Jason gave a manly shrug and walked into the hotel suite with as much dignity as he could muster, his pajamas drooping from beneath his overcoat.

"G'nite, Blackjack," he said.

"Good-night, Jason," said the man, relieved to have unloaded his charge.

Jason gave me a sheepish look as he got into bed next to Valentine. He knew I understood the reason why he was home. Jason was an habitual bed wetter. Sleeping over would be a problem with him until he was several years older. When he was eight Jason underwent a special program to stop bed wetting. It involved flashing lights and ringing bells triggered by wires beneath the mattress at the first drop of urine. But after a few nights Jason slept through the light show. I would come in and take him to the bathroom while the electric cacophony went full blast.

He also fell victim to chronic asthma attacks, which he suffered from infancy. These stopped at about eight or nine, at the same time his bed wetting ceased. Perhaps it was the bell-and-light device or simply a matter of outgrowing the humiliating habit.

Jason regularly attempted to make bondings, especially with dark-haired people. It must have been more difficult than I realized for the boy to find himself growing up so dark in a family of light-haired people—blond David, blond me, blond Paul, blond Valentine; damn it, I even had a blond dog. No wonder he loved old black Henry, the Persian cat.

I can still hear the little old man at the cash register in the corner market question me querulously at the sight of my identically dressed sons, perched one on each hip. "Mother," he asked, "why is one so blond and one so dark?"

"Because one is adopted," I said brightly in my let's-keep-everything-out-in-the-open idealistic attitude. Well, it was okay for me. It was okay for Val and it was okay for Paul. It was even okay for David after he had gone off to live in New York with his new wife. Now I wonder if it was okay for Jason. The romantic family portrait I tried so hard to create just didn't work out with everything and everyone behaving and feeling the way I thought they should. The characters in my play all had feelings, thoughts, and values of their own.

Like me, David completely accepted the fact that Jason would meld in seamlessly with his brothers. His feelings for Jason were identical to his feelings for Paul and Valentine. Naïvely, we thought love was enough and that Jason would automatically fall in with our ways and become like us.

It was not to be.

7
Portrait

1909

Jack posed stiffly in a suit that smelled of camphor.

"He's lovely," said Elsie. "He looks like Bubbles. You know, the Blue Boy in the picture."

Jack was five and had been chosen by his mother to represent her children, her beauty, her strength, and her future.

Jack was uncomfortable in the borrowed finery, but he stood proudly straight with a solemn face, his brown eyes roguish in spite of his efforts to look serious. He wanted to be dignified, befitting the sailor blouse with its large lace collar and the knickerbockers. He was proud because he clasped a large toy sailboat in his arms, complete with mast, sails, sturdy keel, and rudder.

Jack's heart beat fast and he held the boat reverently. He did not want it to slip from his grasp. It was a rich boy's boat and the sailor suit, although no longer new and holding a musty odor, was definitely a rich boy's outfit. The boots now were another matter. Surely no rich boy would be expected to wear these. They hurt. Really hurt. Jack shifted uncomfortably in them.

"Stand still now, Jackie," said the man with the gray beard, sticking his head out from under the black velvet cloth that draped the large camera perched high on a wooden tripod.

Jack immediately stood more erect. He squared his shoulders in an effort to relieve the prickles of pain caused by holding the heavy wooden boat out in front of him. He hoped it would not be much longer before he was able to study the vessel, maybe even play with it. His mouth smiled in spite of his earnest effort at solemnity. He imagined taking this splendid boat to the water trough where the carriage horses drank thirstily after a hard day's work. He could already hear the awe in his brother Albert's voice when he saw the boat.

"Let me hold it, Jack. Can I? Can I play with it? Can I, please?"

And although Jack already felt possessive about the boat, he knew he would let his brother help him carefully launch it. Jack did not know what lucky chance had singled him out, making him the recipient of all these riches, but it felt good. And he could see the glow in his mother's eyes as she stood with his sister, Elsie, watching him. Sister and mother were rooted to the spot, hardly daring to breathe, probably amazed at how grand he looked, thought Jack.

And what was it Elsie had said? He looked like Bubbles. Jack had also seen a copy of the Gainsborough painting, which hung on the wall of their parlor. A dreamy-eyed boy with blond curls, watching soap bubbles float from his clay pipe up into the air. That boy was wearing a blue velvet suit with a lace collar. Women seemed to think he was lovely, though Jack, until this day, thought he looked more like a girl than a boy. But he was admired.

Jack's flight of fancy was brought to an abrupt halt.

"Watch the birdie!"

Jack looked at the man's hand held in the air beside the

camera. Then, *whoomph. Flash!* Jack yelled, a look of frozen horror on his face. The photographer then strode out, grabbed the boat, and said, "Thank you. Next.

"You can pay my assistant over there, Mrs. Ireland."

Oh, the humiliation. What shame Jack felt to think he had imagined the boat had been given to him. He laughed and joked, covered his hot tears of embarrassment as the toy was carried away.

"Silly boat. Heavy! Phew! I'm glad to put that down. It stinks."

Jack's mother stripped him of the photographer's finery, then redressed him in his own familiar shabby, outgrown clothes. The relief of slipping into his own boots stanched his humiliating tears. His own comfortable, worn-out boots.

Later the portrait of the five-year-old dressed-up boy was framed and displayed on the family piano. Jack Alfred Ireland represented the Ireland children. It took two generations before someone said, while looking at the sepia photograph of the winsome young boy, "Why, look, he's wearing two left boots."

8

Hounslow, Middlesex

1938

As if from a bird's-eye view, I saw my mother's and father's small house. It was as like the others in the immediate vicinity as the neatly laid-out front and back gardens.

From the upstairs rear window, slightly ajar, the neighbors doubtless could hear the childish shrieks and giggles that accompanied the sounds of splashing and the light baritone of John Alfred Ireland who was giving his only daughter a bath. It was an uncommon occurrence because this task usually fell to my mother. It was a special afternoon and Jack was busily bathing his squirming, slippery two-year-old.

With much water-slapping and recitations of "This little piggy went to market," the big, natural sponge was generously employed. A large bar of Lifebuoy toilet soap melted murkily on the bottom of the deep, white-enameled tub.

Finally satisfied, Jack Ireland declared ablutions over. He straightened up with a deep sigh of satisfaction for a job well done, held out his arms, and said, "Come on, Jill, out!"

Whereas I had been reluctant to enter the bathtub, I was

now reluctant to get out. So it was to cries of "No, Daddy. No, Daddy, no," that he carefully lifted me from the soapy, rapidly cooling water.

I clasped him tightly around his neck with sturdy wet arms as he, with large, strong, capable hands, wrapped me up snugly from head to toe in a fluffy bath towel.

Then to my glee, he unceremoniously threw me over his shoulder and carried me like a sack of coal out of the steamy bathroom into the bedroom he shared with my mother. Shrieking and giggling with excitement I was plopped down with a thump on the peacock-blue satin quilt that covered my parents' big double bed. Sitting like a plump white sausage amongst the pillows, my back to the polished walnut headboard, I felt happy, secure, and loved. I had a good view of the room with its cozy fireplace and black iron hearth. There was my mother's kidney-shaped dressing table covered with interesting grown-up things—the tortoise shell-backed hairbrush and mirror set and the cut-glass bowl of pale-pink, sweet-smelling powder. On a small silver tray resting lightly in a crumpled ball was a fine hairnet like a bit of fluff beside the many scattered light-brown hairpins. Oh, it was all special, magical stuff. Mummy's stuff. I liked to pat the soft, furry caterpillarlike hairnets with my curious, pudgy child's fingers.

It smelled so good in that room, a mixture of talcum powder and the familiar aromas of my mother and father, a scent that my inquisitive baby nose always picked up, the odor of their bodies from the intimacy of their bed. It was their nest, this bed, a place where they talked, laughed, and occasionally cried out. It was the heart of the house.

Light sifted directly behind the dressing table from a window beyond which could be seen a flower-filled back garden. A light breeze softly moved the pale-blue curtains, fanning the sweet perfume of lilac into the room. The sunshine etched slowly moving patterns of light on the wall behind the bed.

Daddy's exertions caused beads of perspiration to form on his brow. He sang while briskly toweling me until my two-year-old body was rosy, warm, and dry. I bounced merrily up and down on the mattress as he sang, "When the red, red robin comes bob-bob-bobbin' along."

I loved it when he put his head to one side and sang to me, "Cheer up, cheer up, you sleepy head. Cheer up, cheer up, the sun is red."

"Ch'up, ch'up," I joined in.

He sang so well and knew all the words. And when he didn't know the words, he whistled and trilled in a cocky, street-urchin way.

It was the only time I could remember Daddy giving me a bath. I inhaled the essence of the moment, watching him and earnestly storing the memory in the back of my mind in my baby computer.

I would always remember this day and my daddy with his strong, suntanned body, the white slacks, the sleeves of his open-neck shirt rolled back to his biceps in a vain attempt to keep his shirt dry.

He was *my* daddy and I loved him possessively, passionately, innocently sure that life would always be this way. I looked adoringly up into his face. He was so handsome with his strong cheekbones and dark hair over thick brows. His brown eyes shone with loving intelligence and humor. I gazed into them; then, showing off, full of happy confidence, I jumped up and down on the bed. I bounced, singing along, "Ch'up, ch'up, red robin." It was hard to keep my balance on the slippery blue-satin counterpane.

I fell.

Suddenly, with a body-shocking jolt I was in the glare of bright California sunshine. In the blink of an eye I was transported from my childhood home in 1938 in Hounslow, England, to Bel Air, U.S.A., my home in 1985.

I was lying on a lounge chair on the pretty Mediterranean terrace behind the house. Squinting against the sun, I looked into my father's face. He was watching me with large, curious eyes through horn-rimmed spectacles. I knew I had been laughing aloud. I smiled at him sheepishly.

"Hi, Daddy. I just had forty winks. I was dreaming about you."

"*Lo lo lo,*" he said. "*Lo? Lo?*"

He cupped his hand over his ear and I noticed he wasn't wearing his hearing aid.

"Yes, that's right. It's tea time," said I. I kissed him on the top of his head.

My father could no longer speak. He suffered a stroke in 1977. It is a frustrating condition, aphasia. The victim understands everything. But, tragically, he has lost his powers of communication. Struck on the left side of his brain by a blood clot, Daddy tries to write with his left hand, undaunted by the fact that the stroke paralyzed his right arm. But no matter how he tries, his handwriting comes out like ancient Greek. His attempts to speak to us on paper are as garbled and unintelligible as his efforts to verbalize. He is locked into his head, a prisoner within himself, a man with more than eighty years of memories to share. But sadly for us all, he cannot. No afternoons spent with his family sharing do-you-remember-whens. When he tries to relate all the memories, the jokes he loved to tell, we are left with big, sad eyes and *lo lo lo*'s.

But still, life goes on, so I made a pot of tea in the big blue-and-white-tiled kitchen. I set the china teapot on a tray with two white mugs decorated with four-leaf clovers; a jug of milk, sugar bowl, and a plate of chocolate-chip cookies completed the tray.

I carried it carefully into the garden where Daddy sat comfortably in a deck chair overlooking the crystal-clear swimming pool. He was smiling with pleasure, watching a tiny hummingbird drink nectar from deep inside a white, bell-shaped magnolia blossom. It was October in Bel Air and the weather was clement. I observed my father as I served tea. So different from the man who had been playing and singing with me in my dream. That man was young, athletic, quick-witted, and full of life. A man who teased me and made jokes. This man was eighty years old. His hair, although still thick, was completely white.

His body had thickened with age and his right arm was paralyzed. When the arm was not placed in his jacket pocket it swung uselessly at his side, changing the shape of his shoulder and giving his back a vulnerable appearance. In spite of all this my father had not given in. He still was determined to lead an active life. He walked two miles every day and dressed himself with his one good arm. He was fiercely protective of his independence. As for jokes and stories, his inability to communicate never prevented him from trying to hold conversations. This made everyone's life a constant round of Twenty Questions—a game in which, somehow, my father was the smart one. We were treated as infuriating dunces, for we had not mastered the tricky language of *lo lo*.

If my father needed or disapproved of something, he certainly made his feelings clear. On his absolutely best behavior in a restaurant, still acting as master of ceremonies, Daddy would make the fluttering gesture with his fingers against his lips to say simply, "I cannot speak," when the waiter asked for his order. No insisting and *lo lo* here.

However, if he noticed a guest's wineglass was unfilled, then a stern *lo lo* in my mother's direction and his hand indicated the guest who needed attention.

My mother gave card parties once a week in their home in Seaford, Sussex, where they lived in a small bungalow. Friends dropped in to lose their money to wily Jack who could still play a mean game of gin rummy.

His indomitable gallantry was awe-inspiring. But sometimes, as I watched him, it seemed as if my heart were permanently seized in the grip of pain. His efforts were sad to witness. As I poured his tea I realized my feelings were now maternally protective.

I looked at the man so different and yet so much the same as the one who had sung to me in my bath all those long years ago. I let my mind slip back once more to the blue satin counterpane as I wriggled in my father's grasp.

On that day my father had dressed me with awkward masculine fingers. He fastened the small scarlet china buttons on my favorite gray-and-white floral silk dress. Then he gently brushed my hair with Mummy's soft bristle hairbrush. Because it was him, and he didn't know any better, I was able to persuade him to let me wear my best white buckskin party shoes. Daddy put me down on the floor and returned to the bathroom to mop up and empty the bath while I, proudly dressed in my best, maneuvered with great difficulty down the flight of very steep stairs.

The steps were so precipitous that I sat on my bottom and went down on my seat. At the foot of the staircase I came to my feet to find myself in an entry hall. There was a tall hat stand by the front door with a colored glass window through which light shone to brighten the dimness. Then I entered an airy room with floor-to-ceiling French windows, allowing light to fill the space. In a corner was a green screen. I was drawn to it. It was strange; it hadn't been there before.

In its shadow was a tall new baby crib. It was so high I had to pull myself up on tiptoe to see into it. Oh, and I did want to see into it very much. The smell was alluring, warm, and somehow familiar. As I strained to see more clearly the round lump deep inside the crib, I was startled by an unfamiliar and unfriendly female voice.

"You bad girl! You bad girl! Get away from there."

An officious midwife clad in dark green was hovering over me, pulling me roughly away from the crib. I felt guilty. I looked up at her, ashamed at having been so bad. Suddenly there was another voice, just as angry.

"No, she's not a bad girl. Don't you call her that. Come along, Jill, it's all right."

It was my Auntie Edie. She took my hand and led me away. I was still numb with shock, confused. I had only wanted to see my new baby brother.

My mother's older sister, Edith, had been my friend when I was a little girl. Edith never married, having been, I was told, disappointed in love at an early age. However, she went on to become a successful businesswoman. Throughout my teen years Auntie Edie, who was my godmother, supplied me with many luxuries that my mother and father could not have afforded. Beautiful dresses. Expensive shoes. Trips to foreign countries. I loved my Auntie Edie. She was rescuing me from that frightening lady who hovered over the crib.

I went off with my auntie to the kitchen for a biscuit, as cookies are called in England. I heard Daddy enter the other room and speak softly to my mother.

My mother was the youngest of three sisters. She would probably be the first to admit she was not the prettiest. She was, though, the only one to be married. Dorothy Eborn Ireland was slender with beautiful thick hair, shapely legs, and a peaches-and-cream complexion. Mother, like all of the Eborn family, carried the stamp of generations of fair, blue-eyed Anglo-Saxon stock.

The Eborn men were all well over six feet with strong-boned noses. Even the women were tall, apart from my mother, who for some reason ceased growing at the height of five-foot-four. Her five brothers, George, Arthur, Harry, Ernest, and William shared several traits: their voices were loud and confident. They were robust. They were funny. They were quite simply Eborns. It was stamped all over them.

Jack Ireland stood a mere five-foot-eight and was always impressed with the size of his future brothers-in-law, whom he found abnormally large.

One day during their courtship, my mother, in a pretty

summer dress, leaned coquettishly against a wall. She gazed up into Jack's eyes flirtatiously, willingly allowing his masculinity to dominate her, one of his arms braced beside her head. Jack felt as if he had speared a butterfly against a wall. Suddenly a shadow loomed over him.

Jack looked up to see that blotting out the sun was a huge man strolling by. Said Jack, "Are your brothers as tall as him?"

"Oh," said Dorothy innocently, "they're all much taller."

Jack liked to say he shrank in his shoes and prayed the brothers Eborn would approve of him.

Auntie Edie never believed Jack was quite good enough for her sister Dolly. But it was just his touch of the streets that spiked my blood and strengthened my character.

9

Jack and Dolly

1930s

When I was a little girl I always marveled at the affectionate relationship among my Eborn cousins and their fathers, those giant, sandy-haired, blue-eyed men with their Roman noses, easy confidence, and loud booming jocularity. They handled their children with overt love.

It was not unusual for my Uncle Arthur, my mother's middle brother, to say in a loud, clear voice as he lifted his daughter Alma, "Oh, there's no one like my Alma." He would hug her and stroke her head and ask all and sundry, "Isn't she beautiful?"

This never ceased to amaze me as it was so foreign to the behavior of my father. In contrast to those large, relaxed, affable Englishmen, Daddy was small, dark, muscular, and a man of few words. He never told me I was pretty, let alone beautiful. And as for asking the world in general if I were, the whole idea was out of the question. He quite simply was not demonstrative.

I did not wish he would treat me as my uncles did their daughters with their teasy, easy affection. It just wasn't Jack and I knew it. He even disapproved of other people complimenting me. Once at a wedding when a man said, "Jack, Jill's growing quite beautiful," he hushed him up hastily and said, "Don't let her hear you saying that."

It was too late—I'd heard. But the compliment meant nothing to me since it did not have my father's approval and confirmation.

At family gatherings on holidays and at weddings and the like, my father, when the Eborn clan was gathered, seemed to be lost in a forest of large men and tall, handsome women. As indeed was my mother, who was the shortest in her family. Perhaps that's why she was drawn to my father, someone with whom she could see eyeball-to-eyeball. She was not his Dolly—as they called her—she was simply his "Doll."

One day recently, I drew my mother into conversation about the loves and attitudes of the Eborns and Irelands during my parents' courtship in the 1930s.

I asked, "How did you and Daddy meet?"

My mother and I were sipping vodka and tonic, a favorite drink of ours, in my California beach home. She swirled the ice in her glass and said, "We worked for the same firm. I was a cashier at Platt's Grocery. The receipts were kept in a large tray with the different coins and notes set out. I had to count it all and check the cash against the books. One day in the midst of this process a bee flew down my blouse and stung me on the back of my neck. I threw up my hands and, *crash!* all the coins and notes flew into the air."

She laughed at the memory. Her face flushed, perhaps from the vodka.

"Jack, your father, appeared from nowhere and removed the stinger from my neck. He applied some ice and all was well. Jack also picked up the money and we found ourselves face to face on our hands and knees recovering the coins."

"Was that the beginning of your romance?" I asked.

"Not really. I had a boyfriend meeting me after work on his bicycle. His name was Percy. It wasn't a serious romance because my mother never encouraged young men to come courting. Percy never came to my home."

I suggested, "Maybe that's why Auntie Edie and Auntie Ciss never married."

I refilled her glass as she replied, "My mother was quite strict. When a young man did come calling she put a straight-backed chair outside the back door and gave him a magazine to read."

"Did you have many beaux, Mummy?"

"Enough, considering they never got in the house. There was a young man named Leonard Flick who ran a sports business and, of course, Percy, who married another girl."

"Did Daddy get the chair-and-magazine treatment?"

"No. Not Daddy."

Fascinated by this family history, I asked, "What happened when your brothers brought girls home?"

"That rarely happened until the relationship was very serious. That's different, isn't it? It was the daughters she was protecting."

I asked, "Didn't you find the chair outside embarrassing?"

Mummy looked sad. "Yes, I was terribly embarrassed because all the other girls' mothers allowed their young men in the house. My sister Edie was embarrassed too. She knew one lad I thought very nice, a detective sergeant in the police force. But she never brought him home because of the chair policy. He eventually married another girl."

"And Daddy?" I could not see him sitting outside on a chair.

"When Jack Ireland came to visit he entered the house bold as brass. I remember I had given him gold cuff links for his birthday. I think he still has them."

Her face softened as the sun set over the ocean. "I know very little about Jack's past. He was orphaned at an early age and lived with his sister Elsie and his brother-in-law, Bill Davis, through most of his growing-up and teenage years. Still, when I met him he was a generous, happy-go-lucky sort of chap."

"How did he propose?"

"I don't remember him doing that," my mother replied.

"Come on, Mummy, he must have said something."

"Weelll," she said, taking a generous belt of vodka. "It was just before Christmas at Grandma's house and Jack asked if I would like to have an engagement ring as a Christmas present."

"Did you want one?" I asked.

"I guess I did, because I got one," was her response.

"And that's it, Mother?"

"That's it," she said, finishing her drink.

"Had you not married Daddy, would you have continued to work in the store?"

"I think not. I loved children and I might have become a nursemaid. I worked briefly at that before I met your father, and I enjoyed it."

"Did you continue to work after you married Daddy?"

"Yes. Jack and I enjoyed working together. We worked hard all week with only Sunday and a half day off during the week. We'd go to see films once a week and take walks in Richmond Park.

"In those days working wives were rather frowned on. People felt your husband should be able to keep you. I liked work because Jack never arrived home until eight o'clock at night. Women were supposed to stay home and knit socks, run the house, and do the shopping."

We both needed a drink after that.

My mother sighed and said, "Your father seldom spoke of his past. He remembered that his was not a close family after his mother died. In his middle years he took his sister, Elsie, to visit their oldest brother, Fred, with whom they had lost contact years earlier. They knocked on the door and when Fred appeared your father said, 'How do you do. I'm your brother Jack.'

"And your uncle Fred replied, 'And is this your wife?'

"'No,' your father said. 'This is your sister Elsie.'"

My mother laughed and said it was high time she went to bed. After she retired I sat thinking how my father had once told me the same story with a wry smile.

He said, "That's how close we were. We had tea and I never saw Fred again. I think he's dead now, but I'm not sure."

Misfortune struck early in my parents' marriage in the form of illness. At the age of eleven months, I, their firstborn child, contracted a rare blood disease accompanied by high fevers and vomiting.

My mother took me to a large children's hospital in London where she was told that I would have to remain because little was known about the malady. Sadly, Dorothy left her little girl behind isolated in a glass case.

Hands were encased in rubber gloves to feed, bathe, and change me. Nurses attempted to placate the frightened child. But they did not.

The sense of loss, the loneliness and isolation were more than my little girl's mind could absorb. However, after many days, I came to accept that this was what life had become. I had been abandoned.

My mother remembers standing, looking at me through the glass cage. I lifted my arms and called, "Mama!"

My mother waved and tapped her fingers on the pane. She blew kisses.

"Hello, Jill. Hello, Jilly."

Seeing that my mother was not going to take me from the prison, I began to wail. My grief returned in all its majestic proportions. My mother watched me crying as long as she could before sadly turning and walking away. She caught the train for the long ride back to the suburb of Hounslow. She would not show herself again for several weeks. The experience was too upsetting for the baby, she told herself.

At home, Jack put away the high chair and pram to spare his wife the constant reminders of their absent little daughter. Dorothy continued to visit me, taking pains to keep out of my sight to avoid the outburst of tears and grief.

Many weeks later Jack and Dolly were allowed to bring their child home again.

10

Jack and Jill

1940s

As I was growing up, my father was a vivid but somewhat shadowy figure. He was always going to work with a cheery good-bye, or coming home from work to eat his dinner as I was going to bed. My brother and I would have dinner at an earlier hour, usually the same meal that had been prepared for my father. When faced with my own supper, I had little appetite and pushed the food around on my plate with a fork in desultory fashion.

When Daddy sat down to eat his dinner with my mother, the same food suddenly appeared most appetizing and appealing. Clad in my dressing gown, nightgown, and slippers, I would pull up a chair beside Daddy and proceed to watch him enjoy his meal. Daddy covered his food with pepper, something I was not allowed to do or didn't want to do.

Just before Daddy finished, I would say, "Can I have some, Daddy?" and he would give me a teaspoon and let me finish what was on his plate. It tasted wonderful, hot and peppery, quite different from the fare I had been given earlier.

"Jill, you don't want that," my mother would say.

Oh, but I did. Those few teaspoons donated by Daddy tasted better than anything I had eaten in my life. Then it was off to bed with me.

I loved my father, but I cannot say we were close. Most of our relationship went on in my imagination. I was most sympathetic toward him at all times and excused any transgressions.

From the time I was three, I was enrolled in ballet school and performed in the recitals that seemed to come around at least every few months, and the big one at Christmas. My father must not have enjoyed them because he seldom turned up. They pleased my mother, however, who urged me on to greater endeavors.

I was aware that my father did not share my mother's interest and I never really expected him to be in the audience. Occasionally he would appear, although he never commented on my performance.

Once I asked my mother, "What did Daddy say?"

"I think your father believes you always try to do something that's too difficult," my mother replied.

Try as I might to get my mother to elaborate on the remark, she could not or would not. It left me, though, with a feeling that my performance wasn't quite as good as my father would like to have seen it.

My father liked women. Although I never had any substantiation, I remember one night being awakened from a sound sleep by my mother, saying, "Jill, I want you to go round to that woman's house and ask them to tell your father not to stay there so late." She was visibly upset to my ten-year-old eyes. And now with the eyes of a mature woman I can see she must have been quite desperate to awaken her daughter in the middle of the night. Desperate, lonely, and very, very angry.

She needed someone to talk to and I was the only female in the vicinity.

"I'll do it, Mummy," I said. "When do you want me to go?"

"First thing in the morning," she said.

"Okay."

My poor mother, I realize now the hours had crept by so slowly, trapped as she was in her home with two young children she couldn't leave, while my father was out gallivanting, singing and dancing and who knows what else at the home of a person my mother referred to as "that woman."

I went to sleep again long before my roving father returned. So I was not witness to what must have been quite a reconciliation. I only remember the following morning reporting earnestly to my mother, ready for active duty. "Do you want me to go round to that lady's house now?" I asked.

"No," said my mother airily. "He came in and made a fuss of me. It's all over now. Forget about it."

But of course I didn't. To this day I wonder whose home it was and if he ever went back.

My father's maternal grandfather was named Malachi Isles. According to my cousin Beryl's husband, an Irishman named Dennis Williams, Malachi is an Irish name, which conflicts with my father's theory that such a dark-haired, olive-skinned family must have been of Italian origin.

I grew up under the impression that I was part Italian on my father's side. A strange combination, I am. One part swarthy, dark, passionate, Latinate, and the other tall, blond, blue-eyed Anglo-Saxon. I look like my mother's side of the family, but I believe I get my nature from my father. And it has been said that if my hands were tied behind my back I could no longer speak.

Jack's first real job was as a cinema attendant—or an usher as they are called today. The rest of his working life was spent in the grocery trade.

He worked his way up through various managerial positions in a large chain of stores. He took great pride in selecting wines and gourmet foods. At Christmastime he made sure well-plucked chickens of the finest quality were delivered to his customers. Each holiday season Daddy rolled up his sleeves and pitched in beside his workmen, plucking feathers until his fingers were raw.

Daddy was a hard-working, hard-drinking, two-fisted man's man. He liked women, singing, and dancing. He was the sort who always picked up the check. He never lost his artistic bent and through the years painted in oils on canvas. He often helped with my homework by illustrating my compositions, thus raising my grades.

Daddy loved parties and I remember we attended many as a family. I also recall when the music started my father danced with all the women and young girls. There never was a wallflower when Jack Ireland was around.

He inevitably asked me to dance at parties. I learned a complicated foxtrot while gliding across the floor, his hand placed squarely in the middle of my back, often accidentally raising my skirt a little higher than my girlish modesty wished. We danced rather gracefully despite my silver ankle-strapped wedgies. He was fun to be with. He truly knew how to live in the moment.

My father was always an emotional man. He wept while I was doing my best to enter this world. My mother was with the midwife in her bedroom. I was in my mother trying to get out. My father was downstairs crying and making such a noise that my mother sent word for him to go out for a walk.

"For goodness sake, Jack, you're making more noise than I am. Anyone would think you were having the baby. Go out for a walk, and by the time you come back it will be all over."

So he did.

When he returned I was waiting for him.

My parents were a passionate and somewhat noisy

couple. They had many spats. Daddy had, and still has, a quick temper, and although he never struck my mother, his voice was loud and mighty. His thundering frightened me because he often seemed out of control when in the grip of one of his rages. No matter how angry, however, he was never heard to utter a profanity or vulgarity. It would never have occurred to him to do so.

One dinnertime my parents, brother John, and myself were at table while father honed a large carving knife along an ivory-handled sharpening steel in preparation for carving a Sunday roast beef. He suddenly became enraged by something my mother said. I was only about eight and Mummy's remark had gone over my head. But my father's reaction did not.

He raised his fist, holding the knife in the air. Since I was sitting on his right, the knife appeared to be poised in his trembling hand directly over my head. Daddy's whole body shook with anger.

My mother said softly, "Jack, don't."

Fighting back tears of fear, I looked up at my father. "Daddy, please," I said.

My father stood there a moment longer in the grip of his terrible rage. Then he slammed the knife down on the table and marched from the room. I can remember no more. But the image of my father at that moment remains with me, as it will, I know, forever.

My father's terrible temper was well known and much feared by his staff at Platt's Stores, of which he was general manager.

But he was popular with the men and women who worked for him. Jack was a most attractive man with a jaunty style. He dressed elegantly. He wore well-cut jackets, smart suits, polished shoes, and a felt trilby hat, never forgetting to remove it when encountering a lady or entering a building. He had automatic good manners. When we were out together I became accustomed to his walking on the side closest to the roadway. When we crossed a street, on reflex once again, he would wait to allow me to take the inside path. He had a funny little whistle. No tune at all really, just a happy chirping sound to accompany him when he ran up and down the stairs of our house or while working in the garden, which he loved very much.

My father enjoyed helping people. He used his strength, spending it generously, helping build a wall, mixing concrete, painting a house, laying a carpet. Since he could never leave a job half done, whoever involved Jack Ireland in a project was a lucky man. He worked rapidly, then dripping with perspiration he would breathe a sigh of relief and go home to bathe and have his dinner.

11

Sacked

August 1969

Dorothy's eyes sparkled when she looked out the window to see Jack's car pull into the driveway.

She hurried quickly down the stairs to meet her husband and approached him for their customary greeting kiss. In all the years of their marriage Jack had never failed to kiss her good-bye on leaving the house and kiss her again on his return.

But this day he came in, walked straight into the sitting room, and sat down in his chair with a thump. He looked at her with a strange expression in his eyes and said, "Give me a drink."

Dorothy's spirits fell. She studied her husband. "What's happened?" she asked.

Jack stared at her in disbelief. "They sacked me. Three weeks before my pension, they sacked me."

"Oh, my God."

Dorothy sank down on the settee, all the pleasure draining from her.

Jack's face was ashen.

"I think we'd both better have a drink," she said. "I can't believe they've done this to you after all these years. Does this mean we won't get the pension?"

Jack nodded.

"We'll have to sell the house," said Dorothy. "How will we manage? And what about the car? The company car?"

"They'll take that back," said Jack. "It seems they're closing down the firm and they're laying off everyone. I'm the first to go because I would have got the biggest pension, being the general manager."

Jack Ireland, through dint of hard work and long hours, had risen over the years in the chain of Platt's grocery stores from stock clerk to manager of the entire chain. Now he found himself callously cast aside, a trauma that would soon ruin his health, although it never defeated his spirit.

The two sat in their comfortable, attractive, hard-won drawing room. This, too, would have to go. They would not be able to afford to live in the same style now—not without Jack's pension.

Dorothy felt tears begin. Then she looked at her husband. He seemed defeated and ashamed. It's not fair, she thought. It's not his fault. He's worked so hard for those people all these years.

"C'mon, Jack," she said. "We're going out tonight anyway. Your suit's ready. Come upstairs."

The two drinks had done their job. The color returned to Jack's face and an appreciative twinkle was in Dorothy's eyes as he looked at his wife in her new dress.

"That's nice," he said.

Dorothy smiled flirtatiously. "Come on, old chap, let's get you ready. We'll have another little drink while you dress."

She began to sing:

Another little drink,
Another little drink,
Another little drink wouldn't do us any harm.

They went to a dinner-dance that night resplendent, he in his dark suit and she in her evening gown. They carried on the evening just as they had planned, not telling their friends the bad news that had befallen them. But it was the end of an era for Jack and Dorothy Ireland, the end of Jack's good health. From that day onward he was to suffer ulcerated colitis and Crohn's disease. He underwent a colostomy, three intestinal surgeries, a trio of heart attacks, open-heart surgery involving five bypasses, and subsequently a series of strokes.

12
David and Jill

1963–1967

I had always thought that if anything should happen to my marriage, David and I would remain friends. Close friends. There was too much affection and friendship between us for it to go any other way. That's what I thought.

I paid no heed to a solemn remark uttered by David early in our marriage. He said if anything happened to us, he would never see me or our child again. I hadn't taken him seriously. No one would do that to his own flesh and blood.

Five years later we were facing the end of our marriage.

What we both wanted sincerely was to stay together and to rear our children. There was a song popular at that time with a refrain that ran "There's a lot of love between us. Hang on, hang on, hang on to what we've got." But we could not.

I tried to hang on and I know David did. But there was a far stronger force in the triangle. I tried to hold on to both and when it became obvious I could not keep the marriage going, I tried to hang on to David as my friend and father of my children. But I couldn't cling to that either.

While he lived with the children, David was an attentive, tender, and loving father. He was also busy with his career.

After we separated, David met and fell in love with a New York model named Katherine Carpenter.

David was in Rome at the height of his TV fame in "The Man from U.N.C.L.E." Katherine was with him. During a press conference—without informing me so that I could prepare the children—he announced we were getting a divorce. He may not have done this thoughtlessly, and, knowing the press as I do, he could easily have been taken off guard by an unexpected question. Nevertheless, his announcement appeared on television and the children, who were watching with their nanny, learned in this blunt fashion that their parents were divorcing.

Paul, who had greeted the sight of his father on the screen with excitement, was old enough to understand the consequences of what was said.

When I came home from work, the seven-year-old Paul questioned me closely. I told him. "It doesn't mean that Daddy doesn't love you. He loves you very much. It has nothing to do with your life with Daddy."

Paul cried and said, "But I won't be Paul McCallum anymore. Now I'll be Paul Ireland."

"You'll always be Paul McCallum and Daddy will always be your daddy."

I'm afraid I persisted with this line of reason with all three boys long after it became apparent that to all intents and purposes, Daddy would be a daddy-in-absentia and the fathering would be left to Mommy's new husband.

David and Katherine eventually married and moved to Manhattan, putting three thousand miles between them and the boys. He saw his sons on weekends when he lived in Los Angeles. When he moved to New York, he flew them East now and then, but the visits grew increasingly infrequent.

His new wife presented him with a son and a daughter.

He had a new family and new obligations. He knew his sons were being financially well cared for and that they had a strong father figure in Charlie. So, like a will-o'-the-wisp, David gradually faded from their lives. There were letters at Christmas and on birthdays written in the large, bold hand of his wife, Katherine, and the odd postcard and letter from Daddy in David's handwriting. Once in a while, when work brought him to Los Angeles, he took the boys to dinner.

All the boys called David *Daddy*. Now it became a rarely used word, causing Paul, in particular, much grief and sadness. Val, who never knew when or if his daddy would turn up, remained characteristically optimistic. He hoped for the best and wrote postcards to David reading, "Dear Daddy, I miss you."

Jason was just coming to terms with the word *adoption* and what it really meant—that he once had another mother and father who for reasons of their own had left him.

Now, it seemed to Jason, it had happened again. He clung to me and Charlie steadfastly. Having lost two fathers, he was determined he should not lose a third.

None of the boys ever called Charlie *Daddy*. They already had a daddy. Jason called Charlie Dad a few times, but Charlie had two natural children who called him Dad, so that didn't work too well either.

In spite of all this, Charlie did gather the clan together and the children—Suzanne, Paul, Tony, Jason, and Valentine —came to think of themselves as a family, of which Charlie was the paterfamilias.

He made the rules, paid for their schooling and clothing. He meted the punishment and supplied the rewards. He was not shy to tell them he loved them and he made it clear what kind of a man he was, giving the boys a strong role model. They became his friends and companions.

13

Bronsons

1968

As Charlie's role in our family relationship became dominant, life changed dramatically for my sons and myself.

Charlie daily visited my happy Hollywood Hills home, roughhousing with the boys, driving them to the park and Disneyland.

The boys enjoyed Charlie. Valentine and Jason could not remember when he was not in their lives. From the first, Jason loved Charlie with his hair as dark as his own. And his hard, strong muscles. Jason wanted to be like Charlie when he grew up. He wanted a voice like Charlie's. It was different from any voice he knew, deep, yet with a soft purr. Charlie used to pick up the boys, toss them high, then wrestle with them on the floor, rolling over and over until the boys' heads spun and their sides ached with laughing.

Charlie gave good presents, too. Birthdays, Christmas, and in-between times. Tricycles and small trucks. Cars and balls. Jason loved trucks. As the boys grew, so did their love for Charlie.

While I was married to David and in love with Charlie,

I did everything in my power to keep my life going just the way it was, keeping David and the children intact while tenaciously trying to hold on to Charlie, to give him enough love and attention to keep him satisfied, to stop him from searching for another woman who might be there all the time. I ran from pillar to post, spending time with Charlie, cooking him little meals, running to his house, cleaning it for him at times.

Once Charlie was ill with bronchitis. He lay in his bed in a delirium. I took care of six-week-old Valentine, Jason, and Paul, then left them in the care of my housekeeper and rushed to Charlie's house to check on his fever and persuade him to eat.

His bed was situated in the middle of the room in front of a fireplace in which we kept a fire burning most of the time. It was November and cold for California. I noticed the hearth was filled with cinders and dust from previous fires and that inhaling them might make Charlie's fever worse. So while he slept I found a small dustpan and brush and laboriously swept up the ashes and deposited them in a trash bin at the back of the house. My labors took an hour and many trips.

Then I set new logs in preparation for the evening's blaze when Charlie awoke from his feverish sleep.

"What have you been doing, baby?"

"I've cleaned your grate," I said proudly.

I was rather black, the soot having spread to my blouse and smudged my face.

"Good heavens, how did you do it?" he asked.

"I used the little brush and pan there."

Despite his illness, Charlie laughed. "Don't you know all you had to do is sweep the debris through that hole in the back of the fireplace? It only takes a couple of minutes."

I was angry and embarrassed. I'd never lived in a house in England with such a contraption. "You mean I could have just swept it through the floor? Where does it go?"

"Damned if I know, baby, but you sure didn't have to do it your way." He laughed and added, "Thank you, my little housewife."

We lighted the fire. I fed him the casserole I had made and scurried back home to my other life where I found my husband David. Then I cooked a casserole for him.

It seemed the nicer I was to Charlie, the nicer I was to David to make up for it, to ease my guilt. And the better I treated David, the better I was to Charlie. The whole thing was very exhausting. I was torn between them.

David offered me security. He was the father of my children. He was my background, the memories of my childhood in England. He knew where Swan Walk was in Richmond where I strolled as a little girl. We had mutual friends. Our backgrounds were compatible.

This broody Slavic Russian Buchinsky, now Bronson, with whom I had fallen in love was the complete opposite of my husband. But the pull was irresistible.

In restrospect, I think I would have been extraordinarily happy could I have kept David—my children would have their father—and Charlie. And later having Zuleika with Charlie. I could have been happily married to two men and my children could have enjoyed two fathers. What one offered, the other did not, and vice versa. Zuleika could have drawn us all together. More of Zuleika, my daughter with Charlie, later.

If, then, I could have accepted David's new wife, Katherine, to my bosom and their children, whom I loved on sight, I think life would have been well arranged.

Charlie used to say, "You're like a woman on a trapeze. You swing madly to and fro saying, 'Catch me! Catch me!' Well, I'm saying I will catch you. I'm going to catch you. Let go. Let go."

I finally did, and I didn't fall. Charlie caught me. But there were moments when the trip from one trapeze to the other was heartbreaking, full of tears and sadness, wistfulness and, briefly, bitterness. Eventually, David and I could embrace as friends. David and his daughter Sophie have met my children. And I have met Katherine, Sophie, and their son Peter. I have a genuine affection for them all.

My three boys loved to visit Charlie at his home because Charlie's two children would be there. Jason got to play with Tony, two years his senior. He felt passionately about Tony. His chest filled with excitement whenever he saw Charlie's only son. He would scream his name jubilantly, "Tony! Tony! Tony!"

Tony liked Jason but did not share his adoration. Tony *did* like being adored, worshiped almost. Tony's hair was as black as Jason's. His body was strong and athletic like his father's. When the children were out together, it was Jason and Tony who were taken for brothers. Both were presumed to be Charlie's sons. Jason loved the feeling of belonging. I noticed Tony found it confusing. His father was his. He was his *only* son. Jason bothered him with his wild behavior and demanding, passionate affection for his father and for himself. He would rather play with Valentine or Paul. But since it was only on weekends, Tony put up with it.

Suzanne, five years older than Jason, liked the boy. His energy matched her own and brought out the maternal instincts that sibling rivalry inhibited her from displaying for her own brother.

Looking back, I think Jason saw his chance to blend into a normal family setting inconspicuously the day I married Charlie with his two dark-haired children. Now Paul and Valentine, my two Englishmen, were in the minority.

I saw the potential for jealousy between Tony and Jason, who felt my protection and, under this mantle strained harder to get closer to Charlie and Tony. He yearned for their love, that missing chemistry he had lost along with his heritage the day he was born. He stubbornly decided he wanted that intrinsic bonding with these two dark, male people. He needed their love and approval.

"I want to be Tony's slave," he told me.

Horrified, I explained, "No you don't, Jason. You don't want ever to be anybody's slave."

"I want to be Tony's," Jason answered darkly.

Until the time we merged the Bronson and McCallum children, Jason had experienced only love in his home. Paul and Valentine loved him. I could see that it both surprised and hurt him that the boy who was to become his new older brother did not treat him with the same unconditional love and understanding. But there was nothing I could do about it. I hoped time would ameliorate the situation. Tony needed time to adjust to the boys who would soon be his three new siblings.

Tony's rejection of his hero worship hurt Jason deeply. But in those days Jason ran through his pain, whooping and hollering, distracting himself with constant activity and mischief.

It was only later that Jason found dark and more dangerous ways to mask his primordial anxiety and feelings of inadequacy.

Charlie had made it clear from the beginning that he and his wife, Harriet, did not have a happy marriage. They had been drifting apart for a long time when I met the man who was to become my second husband.

Even before I became his stepmother, young Tony was not having an easy time. That summer Harriet had sent Tony and Suzanne to a camp in the mountains above Palm Springs. Tony was too young for the camp, but Harriet prevailed on the director and they took him in.

While the children were at camp Harriet sold the house the Bronson family had lived in, along with the furniture; the children's beds, desks, everything. Tony, six, and Suzanne, thirteen, never again saw their possessions or the house in which they were reared. Harriet moved into an apartment that did not allow children.

Charlie and I visited the camp on weekends. Tony was

obviously in trouble. Suzanne, tense and defensive, seemed to enjoy camp life somewhat. Tony, being so much younger than the other campers, was unhappy. On one visit I took him a bag of cookies. He ate them like a young wolf. There were dark circles beneath his huge brown eyes. Tony was so miserable he developed a nervous tic, a rapid blinking of his eyes.

He lay down on the grass beneath a big shade tree. I placed his head on my lap and stroked the hair from his brow. Suzanne left a group of girls on the volleyball court and sat beside us. She was glad to see Tony had devoured the cookies, saying he had hardly eaten since he arrived in camp.

"What's more," she said, "he won't sit down at the table at mealtimes. He just stands there."

I wanted to take Tony home with us, but Harriet had custody. Our hands were tied. Poor Charlie, fiercely paternal, fretted and worried about his children. He asked Suzanne to take care of Tony and she did her best. The difference in their ages placed them in separate groups. They ate at different times and slept in different cabins. Tony became disturbed that summer and it would be many years before he lost his nervous tic.

During that busy, traumatic summer of 1968, prior to my marriage to Charlie, we looked for a house that would accommodate a family of seven. Happily for us, Harriet relinquished custody and Suzanne and Tony would live with us. Charlie insisted, despite David's wishes, that Paul should not attend boarding school, so my eldest, too, would be part of our new beginning as a family.

My friend Maggie Longhurst visited me from England at the Hollywood house. Maggie is that rarest of English avis, a blithe gentlewoman of bohemian tastes, amusing and artfully clever. She was the best of companions and every day we met with Charlie and a real-estate agent who showed us houses. It was all unreal. I was twenty-nine and just untangled legally from my marriage to David. For the time being

I still had total control over my children: Paul eight, Jason four, and Valentine, three. We were a close-knit family, a matriarchy.

Eventually, we were shown a bastion of a house on Udine Way, a quiet cul-de-sac in Bel Air. It was nothing less than a mansion, albeit shabby and rundown—otherwise Charlie could never have afforded it.

It rose imposingly high above the street behind a fenced and curved driveway, towering three stories high. It contained twelve bedrooms, a dozen baths, servants' quarters, library, an immense basement with phalanxes of furnaces, soaring, vaulted ceilings in sitting rooms and dining room, a butler's pantry, broad corridors the length of bowling alleys, nooks and crannies aplenty for curious young children.

The house was huge, hollow, and empty, and it echoed with the cries and howls of the children, who roared through the rooms playing hide and seek, shouting from one floor to the other. It was as if the five of them had been turned loose in an abandoned castle.

The back garden and terrace included a sweep of lawn, which would later boast a sparkling blue swimming pool overlooking the endless undulations of the emerald fairways of the Bel Air Country Club.

It was, Charlie decided, a perfect house for all of us once we were married. It was large enough for the family, large enough to give me a headache for twenty years.

The great, gray edifice was in sharp contrast to the cozy, four-level hillside home in which I had lived with my boys. The house on Udine had a definitely male personality, demanding, domineering. It was, and remains, a powerful building. In a sense it became my master and I would serve it faithfully in the years ahead, furnishing each room with love and care, hiring servants to burnish the hardware, woodwork, and glass.

The house could be intimidating, infuriating, and sometimes almost vengeful. Even as Charlie arranged to purchase the place, I experienced pangs of anxiety. I saw myself as a chatelaine, toting a heavy iron ring of keys at my waist while making sure the linens were aired correctly in the cupboards and that all was well with my lord and master, Mr. Bel Air, or Lord Bel Air as it eventually became after years of polishing brass, decorating, painting, and upgrading.

At the end of that summer, although we weren't married, I moved into the fortress with my children and Suzanne and Tony.

The prospect of running the large house with one elderly housekeeper and no real staff to speak of was frightening, as was taking on the responsibility for two more children.

After seven days, my warm, capable housekeeper, Effie, who had come with me and the boys from the Hollywood house, left, saying she wished me luck but it was all too much for her. Effie knew that to preserve her health and sanity, she could not continue to work in that huge domain, helping me care for what had become a pack of wild children and their numerous school friends, who often swelled the ranks to a dozen or more.

As she left, I detected a note of compassion. "Good-bye, Mrs. McCal . . . Mrs. Bronson—take care of yourself. You know what I mean."

I watched her departure with a heavy heart. I was losing the last of my mainstays, the only person apart from myself who could remember how tranquil, warm, and safe life had been with the three boys, my cat, and two dogs.

Also in the first week, Gregory, our basset hound, lolloped off over the golf course, pausing briefly on a hilltop to look back at what must have looked like the sinking *Titanic*. Gregory shook his head mournfully and continued on his way, never to be seen again. It was a long time before we gave up on the thought of finding him. We only hoped Gregory found greener pastures.

Thereafter, it was difficult to find and keep staff at the salary we could afford to pay, people prepared to tackle such an intimidating brood and even more intimidating lord and master. It amounted to running a small hotel—fifteen sets of sheets, towels, bedrooms to be cleaned, not to mention twenty-one meals a day for a family with five notoriously picky eaters.

Reeling from the impact of my new life, I could not set a date for the wedding. I was simply too frightened. Finally, my business manager Larry Martindale and Charlie cornered me in the study of the house and reminded me I was living with Charlie's furniture, his children, and in his home. Didn't I think it was time I set a date, since the poor man was living in an empty bachelor's house, sleeping on the floor.

I said I would let them know. Then I went into the back garden. A friend, Marcia Borie, unexpectedly arrived for a visit and found me in a small puddle of my own tears, head down in the fetal position. She says to this day she remembers the sight.

I looked up at her and said, "I'm so frightened. It's all so overwhelming. I don't think I want to get married again."

Marcia looked around and said, "It's a bit late, kid."

Three days later Charlie and I went to Santa Monica City Hall with all five children and Marcia as a witness. After the ceremony we returned to the mansion on Udine to paint the sitting room.

From the moment I married Charlie and was made the mistress of his house and mother of his children, I was forced to play grownup while most of me was still dying to be one of the children and have fun.

The mantle of motherhood in my new marriage was a heavy one.

For the first several months life was a monstrous game of hide and seek with five children disappearing for hours at a time in different caverns and maws of the great house, disembodied voices, rampaging footfalls, cries and giggles. Their explorations were endless. Then, emboldened by their successes at independence indoors, the youngsters pioneered the fairways and bunkers and copses of trees and shrubs of the country club. It seemed Charlie and I devoted all our time to individual search forays for missing kids, rounding them up for meals, school, and piano lessons.

It was like being a flight controller in a radar tower. I never relaxed. My senses were always alert, my eyes on each child, looking for trouble. I was on ready-reserve at all times, prepared to step in. It was a good thing I was young.

My days of freedom, brief as they were, were definitely over.

A good deal was expected from me as a wife and mother. I tried to prove equal to the task, which I realize now required a staff of mothers, not just one. Instead of going with the flow I decided to become a perfect parent. This meant complete control. Otherwise how could I run things perfectly? Since Charlie also sought total control—to have things go the way he thought they should—we were never completely free of tension.

There is fifteen years' difference in Charlie's and my ages. Our backgrounds, upbringing, and values were at odds. But we had one thing in common. Love. We loved each other and our children. I literally would have killed for them . . . even Charlie would not have been spared.

Throughout those early years I marveled that we achieved all that we did. Charlie's career soared. I worked. We reared the children. I gave birth to Zuleika and took in another child, Katrina. We all survived.

Jason was the only serious casualty, an innocent bystander, shot by the stray bullets of decisions made years before he was born—marriages that did not work out, concepts of child-rearing passed on from different eras and cultures from diverse parts on the map.

Jason's problems multiplied when he entered school. It was then Charlie and I learned he suffered from dyslexia, complicated by hyperkinesia. To such children touch is of major importance; it is the one sense on which they are able to rely. They must touch objects, feel textures. Jason felt doorknobs, legs of chairs, fabric, ornaments, a habit he has carried throughout his life.

Jason's dyslexia meant he could no longer go to school with Valentine. While they attended the Belagio School in Bel Air they were in the same class. The teacher observed she had never seen brothers so close or so loving.

Jason was enrolled in a special school for children with learning disorders, the Lawrence School in the San Fernando Valley. It was suggested Jason take the drug Ritalin, which has a calming effect on hyperkinetic children. His doctor said Jason would probably settle down and do better school work and the drug would not harm him.

It has been learned since that Ritalin can have lasting deleterious effects by intefering with motor responses and shortening attention span. But Jason was given Ritalin every day despite his complaints that it made him sick.

It was administered by the governess in the morning at home and by a teacher at school in the afternoon.

He was told by teachers, doctors, governesses, Charlie, and me: "Take the pills, Jason. They will make you less restless. They will calm you down so you will be able to learn better at school."

And Jason, eager to do well, to match his brothers, took the pills.

It was at the Lawrence School that Jason met his best friend, Cory Greenfield. They became inseparable. They were also in trouble most of the time. Trouble with a capital *T* to the bus drivers and teachers. They were never allowed to sit together in class. I was told, as was Cory's mother Sharon, "Cory Greenfield is a very nice boy. Jason McCallum is a very nice boy. But together they incite each other to great mischief. They should never be allowed to be together."

This was impossible, as they sought each other's company. They regularly threw eggs from the school-bus windows. They mooned passersby when the bus crossed crowded intersections. When they were nine they borrowed Charlie's air rifle and shot out the lights of the Marymount girls' high school. *No* was a word they didn't acknowledge. They were a pair of mavericks who broke the rules.

In school they talked, joked, and laughed, giving teachers endless problems. In spite of this, Charlie, myself, and the rest of the family became fond of Cory. Every summer he accompanied us to our Vermont vacation home. Even in that sylvan setting Cory and Jason would not obey Charlie's rules.

They were told not to dismantle the motorbikes. They were warned about spinning their wheels in the mud. But every day they came into the house drenched and dirty. They were told not to dive onto the tents. But they did. Jason broke the tent post.

The other children were not angels. But the difference was they disobeyed only once or twice. After being reprimanded they fell into line. Jason would not. He never stopped breaking rules. He was funny, wild, a wily free spirit. He got away with everything, at least with me.

My mother once remarked rather tartly, "That boy gets away with murder, Jill."

I laughed her off. "Oh, that's just Jason."

I defended him ferociously. I loved him unconditionally, but he certainly was different.

14

Separation

When Jason was only seven, Charlie and I took Valentine, who at six was the baby of the family, to London on a film location. Charlie suggested leaving Tony, Suzanne, Paul, and Jason at home to avoid missing school.

But Jason and Val had always traveled together with us. It was wrenching for me and Jason, who faced this first separation. I can still see his face. I sat him on my knee in my dressing room and hugged him good-bye.

Jason said, "How long will you be gone, Mom?"

"Not long. About four weeks."

His face was so trusting. How could I leave him?

"Paul is here, Jason. He'll watch out for you."

"Mom," Jason's solemn dark blue eyes turned to me. "Mom, did my father know he sowed his seed?"

I was shocked, amazed at his timing and the almost biblical way he expressed himself. *Sowed his seed.*

I answered him simply: "No, Jason. He didn't."

"Mom, one day I would like to meet my real mother."

"Would you, darling? Why?"

His answer: "I'd like to thank her for not having an abortion."

Charlie had bid his good-bye to Jason and the other children.

"Jason," he called, "let your mother go. She's making us late."

God, if ever there was a moment for decision, this was it. Except the decision had been made. I was going to London with Charlie and Valentine while Charlie made the movie *Twinky*.

I was protecting my marriage and my relationship with Charlie. It meant a great deal to my husband that I accompany him to London. But I was leaving Jason at a moment in his life that was obviously important. This conversation needed more time.

"We're going to miss the plane, Jill."

I hugged Jason tightly.

"I love you, Jason. Remember, Mama loves you very much."

Then I blurted out, "Jason, it's not important how you arrive in this world, in whose body you are delivered. Life is like a party. It's not important what vehicle gets you there. It's what you do when you're there, how much fun you have."

I kissed him and held him. "I love you, my darling little adopted boy. Mama loves you so very, very much."

I hugged him one more time, then put him down and hurried out of the house in tears to join Charlie and Valentine in the waiting black limousine. It would be four weeks before I saw Jason again.

15
Darkness

When Jason's mother left, panic overcame Kier and he regressed to a deeply submerged prenatal memory.

Kier had been sleeping fitfully. The crying he heard for weeks had ceased. They were alone, he and she, lying quietly, but the turmoil surging through her veins was dangerous. Then, with a jolt, she stood up. Kier trembled. She was running, lurching, unheeding of the fetus within her.

Suddenly they hurtled through space, both weightless. He was going to miss his time. He was never going to be born. She was trying to kill him. The impact nearly dislodged him as they fell together down a flight of stairs.

Oh, the bleak darkness. The blackness. His mother had tried to kill him. All Kier could feel was death, darkness, his life slipping away before it began.

"Mother, why? Mother, please. Please, why?"

But Kier had clung to life, remaining fixed to the lining of his mother's womb. The parting was to come later . . .

16
Leach

1970

About six months before the trip to England, Charlie and I had taken into our employ a husband-and-wife couple, Mr. and Mrs. John Leach. He had been a chef on the *Queen Mary* and arrived with excellent references. He was to be our cook, his wife our housekeeper. This couple and Giovana Bartholic were left in charge of the house and our children.

As soon as we were gone, life became a nightmare for the youngsters. John Leach was a little man, slight and wiry, no more than five-foot-five. As if to supplement his height he wore a tall white chef's toque. He may have been small in stature for an adult but he towered over the youngsters. With our departure he became a sadistic tyrant, not only with the children but with his wife and Giovana. Jason and Tony were the smallest and most victimized.

When Charlie and I called the house each day, Leach stood over the children listening to their every word.

One day my old friend Alan Marshall dropped by the house to see how they were doing. What he saw was Suzanne, Paul, and Jason terrified. He knew the boys well enough to realize something was wrong. Alan called me, suggesting I come home immediately, that Jason didn't look at all well. There were dark shadows under his eyes and he had lost weight. Both he and Paul were cowed and uncommunicative.

I flew home at once, accompanied by Maggie Longhurst. We were met at the airport by Leach and an unhappy Jason. He was dressed in a sailor suit and cap I did not recognize. Valentine looked at Jason and laughed.

"Why is he dressed like that, Mom? You look funny, Jason."

Jason did not smile. He didn't even hug me. He just stood beside John Leach and looked at me with his two huge eyes, abject. He seemed incapable of speech. I gave him a hug and tried to jolly him out of what I thought was a coolness because I'd been away. But instinct told me better. The misery came from deep within.

Maggie and I exchanged looks as we followed Leach to the car.

When we reached the house Paul and Suzanne were with Giovana, whom I thought looked rather unkempt, her eyes wild. Suzanne and Paul greeted me and Maggie quietly, almost politely. However, Mrs. Leach welcomed me like a long-lost friend, full of warmth and loving stories about the children and how good they'd been.

"Such good boys," she said, speaking like the ideal nanny from "Upstairs, Downstairs." "And Suzanne, too. Bless her heart. Such a good girl."

The mood was weird, very confusing.

It was nearly dinnertime. Leach seemed to have taken over the role of governess and now he bustled off Valentine and Jason to take a bath while his wife prepared dinner.

Maggie and I went upstairs to unpack, followed by Paul and Suzanne.

"Well, how are you, darlings?" Maggie asked. "It's been ages since I've seen you."

Both children were silent. They did, however, seem to want to stick close to us.

Suddenly Leach appeared with Jason and Val clad in their pajamas. His sleeves were rolled up and an apron covered his trousers. He had given them a bath and he was pleased with his work.

"They're clean as two whistles. I've washed every 'ole in their bodies, madam," he said in his cockney accent.

Maggie's and my eyes shot wide open to make four round *os* as we looked down at the two little boys.

"I beg your pardon?" I asked aghast.

"Is there anything else I can do for you, madam?"

"No, John. Definitely not, thank you."

I drew the boys into the dressing room and closed the door firmly.

Mrs. Leach had cooked a wonderful meal. Giovana, who helped serve, avoided my eyes. I wondered why she was doing Leach's job while he bathed the boys. I would sort that out as soon as possible.

After dinner I put Jason and Val to bed, singing to them and cuddling them both. It was good to have the youngest boys together again. Obviously, they had missed each other and I vowed I would never leave Jason behind in the future.

Back in my bedroom, there was a small tap on the door and ten-year-old Paul entered.

"All right, Mother," he said. "If you want to know what's been happening, I'll tell you. After you left it was horrible around here. John Leach pushed everyone around. He bullied us. He pierced the roof of my mouth with a fork when he forced me to eat. Then he took a plate of spaghetti and mashed it into my face. He pulled a knife on Giovana and also on Tony. I don't know what he does to Jason, but Jason just doesn't talk when Leach's around. He stole Jason's wallet with the money he had been saving for Christmas. He stole twenty dollars, Mom. I think he hits his wife."

"My God, Paul. I'm so sorry. This is terrible. Why didn't you write and tell me?"

"I couldn't, Mom. He took all our mail and read everything we wrote. I couldn't call you. He'd have known."

There was another small knock at the door. Suzanne entered and sat on the bed.

"Suzanne, Paul's telling me all about John."

Suzanne, only thirteen, said, "Yes, we're all scared of him. We sleep together at night for protection. He's a terrible man. He grabbed me and kissed me in an unnatural way."

"God, Suzanne, what do you mean *in an unnatural way?*"

"He *Frenched* me. He did it like the French do."

I was horrified. "You mean he put his tongue in your mouth!"

Suzanne looked embarrassed. "Yes."

Then she raised her head and looked at me, her eyes gleaming with agitation. "He threw Jason across the room and took a knife to Tony. But I kneed him in the balls. Giovana is terrified of him. He fights with his wife all the time and calls her names like 'whore' and 'slut.' One day he slammed the door to Paul's room so hard, three pictures fell off the wall in my room."

I felt sick.

"Paul, Suzanne, you were right to tell me this."

I put my arms around the two children. "Well, I'm home now and I promise he won't ever touch you again. I'm so sorry, darlings."

"It's okay, Mom. I just had to tell you how it was; that's all," said Paul.

I tried not to think, My God, if he put his tongue in Suzanne's mouth, what might he have done to Jason? The child was only seven years old.

"Suzanne?" I asked, "do you think he did anything to Jason in an unnatural way?"

Suzanne looked at me for a long time with a straight,

level look, thinking about it seriously. "I don't know, because Giovana was with Jason most of the time. That's why Leach pulled a knife on Giovana. He was trying to make her quit."

I hugged both children again. "I'm getting rid of that man tomorrow. You can both sleep in here if you like."

"No," Suzanne answered. "I'll go down and sleep in Jason's room with him."

"So will I," said Paul.

I realized what an act of faith that was. To tell me was to invoke Leach's wrath and God knows what else; the menacing butcher knife that he was so fond of polishing while he spoke in threatening tones? Goose bumps rose on my skin.

My heart pounded when I called Charlie in England. Charlie was outraged, furious.

"I'm going to fire him tomorrow, Charlie."

"Don't do it. Wait until I get home. I want to see that son-of-a-bitch."

"Charlie, I can't wait; that could be three weeks. We can't live with this man. He's unbalanced. You should see his eyes. I'm scared of him."

"If he does anything, call the police. But don't get rid of him. I want to get my hands on that fucker."

Charlie was close to exploding and I sympathized, but I could not keep Leach around a minute longer than necessary.

"Is everything all right, madam?" he asked the next morning.

I spoke up as boldly as I could. "No, John," I said. "I'm afraid I have to let you go."

"Is that so, madam," he said menacingly.

"Yes, it is. And what's more I would like you to go this afternoon."

The man's eyes glittered dangerously. He licked his thin lips over and over again and shifted his weight from one foot to the other.

I decided to take the offensive. "And I'll have Jason's

wallet back with the twenty dollars in it. I'm sure you took it for safekeeping, but I would like you to give it to me before you leave or I will call the police."

He was gone within an hour, packed bag and baggage, wife and all.

Jason never saw his twenty dollars again, but sanity had been restored. To this day if anyone brings up his name, the children still react with hostility and hatred.

Charlie will never forget John Leach either. He hopes to run into him. If this should occur, I certainly would not like to be in the man's shoes. Anyone who harms Charlie's family is in big trouble.

17
Family Traditions

1968–1970

There were many good and amusing times while the boys were growing up, especially at Christmastime.

Christmas was a wondrous event when I was a child. It seemed to go on for such a long time. Christmas Eve and the excitement of wrapping packages and going to sleep with an empty sock tied to the bedpost. The sound of the grownups downstairs, playing cards, laughing, my aunts and uncles, my mother and father.

My mother collected the ingredients for our traditional holiday plum pudding for weeks and while she mixed it we all had a stir with the large wooden spoon and made a wish. Daddy worked late Christmas Eve. When he finally came home it was with exuberance and hello to my Uncle Arthur and Auntie Cissy, his wife, and their daughter Alma.

Christmas day, awakening to the silence of the morn and reaching out of the snug warmth of the covers to feel my sock with its inevitable orange in the toe, crinkling paper, bags of nuts. And there in the dim morning light across the room on a chair, lumpy packages tied with ribbons and one year, hung on the wardrobe, a pale-blue organdy party dress with pink-satin ribbons. The prettiest dress I'd ever seen. It was like a dream opening my eyes to behold that dress.

Then later in the day playing with new toys in the sitting room while the adults amused themselves at cards once more. The inevitable walk to the cemetery with Auntie Edie to place flowers on my grandmother's grave, my bare knees turning rosy in the frosty winter air. Knee socks, short coat, new shoes and shiny new hair ribbons, feeling very special, very Christmas Day. Then home again to a big Christmas dinner, always roast beef and plum pudding made by my mother from my grandmother's ancient recipe, written in her handwriting in pencil on yellowing paper.

"Jack's home," my mother would say, delighted. And they would all have a drink. The atmosphere was happy, cheerful, upbeat. Everybody was laughing and kind to each other.

Grownups and children alike sat at a long table set with a white-linen tablecloth. There were bonbons with crackers inside them set beside each place. We pulled out favors and popped charms and wore paper hats. There were blowers that uncurled with a high piping noise.

I was surrounded by a strong sense of family and occasion.

My friends and I made a tradition of going from house to house caroling, then knocking on doors hoping for a penny or a three-penny bit. One year when my brother John was two, my mother called after me, "Jill. Take John along."

With groans and protests, my friends and I turned back to collect my brother. At one house, owned by a schoolteacher and his wife, we sang our hearts out and knocked at the door. At the same time my brother tugged at my coat.

"I've gone poo-poo," he said. The corners of his mouth were turned down.

I knocked at the door again. This house was not forthcoming. There would be no pennies here. Two tears rolled down John's cheeks. With sisterly thoughtfulness I pulled down his knickers, deposited the contents on the red polished tile doorstep, and beat a hasty retreat to the next house.

"God rest ye, merry gentlemen. Let nothing you dismay."

We yelled "Merry Christmas," having left our gift on the doorstep of number 70 Maswell Park Road.

When Charlie and I blended the Bronson and the McCallum broods I attempted to re-create the warm family Christmases of my past. There were certainly enough of us. Five children, Charlie, myself, and usually quite a few friends. We gathered in our large, formal dining room for what became a family tradition, a Christmas concert.

The adults sat down, suitably solemn and anticipatory. Paul was the announcer and linked together the events by playing the piano. Everyone did something. Suzanne, being eldest, started the program with a rendering of "The Skaters' Waltz" on the piano. This was met each year with thunderous applause by the grownups. Next came Tony, who performed conjuring tricks with great verve and intensity, but also with many mistakes and remarks of "Wait a minute. Wait a minute. Now, wait a minute!"

We sat patiently through the conjuring tricks but gave him the same thunderous applause as "The Skaters' Waltz."

Next was Valentine with a guitar almost as large as his small body. He played with childlike virtuosity anything that took his fancy. We all rather enjoyed this.

Jason then stood in the middle of the room gravely facing his audience as Paul played portions of "The Maiden's Prayer" while announcing to the assembled company Jason's barnyard impersonations.

"I was walking down the lane and I saw a rooster, arrgh-arrgh-adoo," crowed Jason in an alarmingly loud voice, throwing back his head to crow at the ceiling, flapping his elbows for wings. One could almost see the feathers sprouting. A few more bars of "The Maiden's Prayer" and Jason segued into "And then as I walked through the field I saw a bull, moo, moo." Jason stamped and pawed the floor menacingly.

"And a cow, baw, baw." More tinkling on the piano and then, "A dog," said Jason, raising his leg on the piano, "Woof, woof."

By now his audience was trying hard not to dissolve in inappropriate mirth. Jason took his impersonations seriously. Sometimes he varied his animals with cars he had seen parked outside along the driveway. "A Mercedes," he would say, hooking his fingers into the corners of his mouth, exposing his teeth, and rounding his eyes for the headlights, and making a fierce sound.

Applause for Jason was tentative as we never knew when he was finished. He was apt to spring back into the center of the floor with one more impersonation that he had forgotten.

The evening's entertainment was rounded out by Paul with a vocal rendering:

Passengers must please refrain
From passing water while the train
Is standing in the station
If you please.
Hoboes passing underneath
Will catch it in their eyes and teeth
And that will not contribute to their ease.

In addition to our Christmas tradition I introduced another tie that bound our clan—*The Good Book* and *The Bad Book*.

Into *The Good Book* were entered all the good deeds the children did during the week. Into *The Bad Book* went the reverse. On pocket-money day the children sat down and I read from both books. Each child was given his allowance and then a dime was deducted for every entry in *The Bad Book* and a dime added for each entry in the *Good*. Allowances were staggered according to age.

Typical *Good Book* entries:

Tony helped clean the bathtub, signed Giovana.
Paul put the boys to bed, signed Mother.

Bad Book:

Suzanne refused to wear her raincoat to school, signed Mother.
Jason pushed Tony in the pool and laughed, signed Giovana.
Valentine ran through the house, signed Charlie.
Tony slammed the front door, signed Charlie.

There were times when Jason quite ran out of pocket money, so Suzanne generously donated some of her good deeds to Jason, thus earning herself another entry in *The Good Book*.

18
Almería

1970

In the early days of our marriage we were a nomadic band of Bronsons, traveling to two or three motion-picture locations a year in such exotic countries as Turkey, Spain, England, France, Italy, and Mexico. Usually we took along our entire clan complete with dogs, a cat, and help.

When I was five months pregnant with Zuleika the family departed for Spain. It would be a happy time for Jason, eight, and Valentine, seven. Paul remained at home with Tony and Suzanne attending school, visiting Spain only during the Easter holiday.

It was the two youngest boys' last days together as "the babies." In a short time they would be "my big boys" and the baby, which was making its presence more evident, would soon displace them as the youngest.

Almería, in the south of Spain on the Mediterranean coast, was relatively undeveloped in those days, which gave the boys freedom to run. Also on hand for roles in the picture was the Dick Van Patten family. Dick's son Vincent, who went on to become a seeded tennis player, was a child actor with some imagination. When Vincent was not working he was making his own film, using his own small movie camera. The two stars, and indeed the entire cast, were Jason and Valentine. They would return after a long day's filming with Vince, the director, covered in black paint, ragged clothes, and artificial blood. They were quite a horrifying sight. It took me some time to clean my tow-headed Indian and my black-haired pirate of the makeup and gore that Vincent had finagled from the makeup and special-effects men.

The three boys were most sincere about their endeavors and quite convinced that they had begun careers of major cinematic proportions. I did wish sometimes that either Jason or Val had been the director instead of a principal character in what was a most mucky movie.

Michael Winner, who was directing the film *Chatto's Land*, in which Charlie was starring, invited the boys to play extras. Once more they were dressed in rags, smeared with black paint, and thrown in with a group of older local gypsy boys who did not take their craft as seriously as did my two thespians.

Charlie did not want to cramp their style or embarrass them, so we waited until the end of the day to visit the location. Me with my large belly artfully draped with an antique Spanish shawl. We were horrified by what we found.

Michael was giving his attention to the action in the foreground. In the background, dirty, ragged, and bloody, were my two sons valiantly trying to be professional while the band of gypsy boys beat the hell out of them every time the word *action* was yelled and the kids in the background were told to play.

Jason matched the gypsies in appearance, and so did flaxen-haired Valentine, transformed after the gypsies had dunked his head in the muck and mire. He was caked with mud, entirely concealing the color of his hair.

The gypsies were bigger, stronger, and without scruples.

Once "action" was sounded, Valentine was flung to the ground, face down, his head ground into the dirt. Then a band of grinning, swarthy boys piled on top. They couldn't understand a word Valentine was saying, nor he them. Jason tried to walk from point A to B as directed, but he himself was under attack from a taller, long-haired boy who ran to hit, trip, and push him. Jason, indoctrinated in show business from birth, knew how important it was that the show must go on, at least until someone called "cut." So he did not defend himself.

I couldn't stand seeing how miserable the boys were. Charlie came to the rescue. He stood up from where we had been sitting inconspicuously. Not waiting for someone to yell "cut," much to the director's amazement, Charlie gave his piercing whistle, one that our family reacts to. Jason heard and turned to hear Charlie yell: "In the mouth, Jason. Hit him in the mouth!"

A look of profound relief came over Jason. He hauled off and landed one on the bigger boy's nose. *Whack!*

Now they were into it, punching, gouging, a street fight. The gang atop Valentine got up to form a circle. I think the baby within me started kicking from my excitement. Suddenly the gypsy boy broke from the circle to run away from Jason, which was a surprise because he was so much bigger. Jason followed in hot pursuit, triumphant to have the boy on the run. But it was just a trick.

When Jason gained on him, the boy hit the ground and rolled in a ball sending Jason flying over his head, as in a Tom and Jerry cartoon. The pack of gypsies were closing in on my stunned boy when once again the piercing whistle sounded. Everything stopped. Charlie stalked out into the battleground and grabbed both boys. "Shake hands; it was a good fight."

Jason glared at the gypsy, who grinned appreciatively. It had been a good fight, but Jason was furious.

"I'da got her, Charlie, if I'd been wearing my good boots."

Jason thought he'd been fighting a big, tough girl because the gypsy had such long, curly hair, and the wardrobe department had dressed him in a long, flowing shirt.

Charlie smiled. "Jason, I know you would. Now shake hands. He's a boy, not a girl."

"Ugly, too," said Jason.

Thankfully, the gypsies couldn't speak English. They shook hands. Charlie waved good-bye and led my sons over to me. I restrained an impulse to hug them to my bosom. I allowed them a dignified exit and we drove back to the hotel.

For their day's work the boys each received the princely sum of twenty dollars. Jason spent it all at the hotel gift shop.

He bought me a ring and matching earrings. He didn't seem to mind that all his earnings went into this gift. He was a tough, masculine little boy and he walked square-shouldered beside me that summer in the streets of Almería, making sure no one bumped me, moving people off the pavement, clearing my way, saying, "Look out. Move. My mother's pregnant."

Several days later our car paused at an intersection. On a corner stood the very gypsy boy, still in rags, who had fought with Jason. He spied his foe in the car and gave a comradely wave.

"Wave back," Charlie told Jason, who obeyed grudgingly.

As we turned the corner, I heard Jason say through clenched teeth, "I still say I could have beaten her if I had been wearing my own boots."

In early July 1971, I returned from Almería eight months pregnant. Charlie had to stay on to finish the movie. Because of my imminent delivery, I chose to go home before I passed the point of no return. Valentine, Jason, and I repaired to Los Angeles via London.

During our brief stop at a hotel near Heathrow Airport, we were joined by my mother and father, who were to travel to California with us for a visit until the baby was born. My mother wanted to be there to see her new grandchild.

A few weeks earlier my father had undergone surgery for fistulas but my mother assured us he had recovered. Once safely in Bel Air I discovered my father's health was not as good as I had been told.

I entered my parents' room one evening unexpectedly to find my mother remaking the four-poster bed in which they slept. I asked why.

My mother looked a bit embarrassed. She said, "Well, I put a plastic pad under the sheet every night. I don't like the staff to see it, so I take it off every morning."

She explained my father had been having heavy night sweats and she didn't want to risk staining the mattress.

"What did the doctors say?" I asked.

"We didn't tell the doctor. It will clear up in a few weeks; it probably has something to do with his surgery. It's been like that since he came home from hospital."

"But, Mother, that just isn't right. Does he run a fever?"

"A what?" she asked.

Florence Nightingale my mother never was.

"A temperature, Mother," I said irritably, rubbing the small of my back, which was beginning to ache with monotonous regularity.

"How would I know if he had a temperature?" she said.

I saw the familiar truculence in her eye. I could tell she was going to be stubborn about this.

"You take his temperature, Mother."

"How would I do that?"

I said, "Oh, for God's sake. With a thermometer."

"Well, I don't have a thermometer, whatever that is," she replied.

I couldn't believe my ears. Now I was bordering on

furious. "Mother, you mean you've reared two children and you've never had a thermometer in the house?"

"Oh, we don't do things that way. We do things *our* way," she said in a patronizing tone.

"Well, for God's sake. I'm amazed. I'm surprised that we survived. I can't believe you don't have a thermometer and you don't know how to take a temperature. I've never heard of such a thing."

"Well, you're alive, aren't you?" she said tartly. "So I suppose I must have done something right."

My temples pounded. I felt the baby inside me stir. "Mother, I am going to bring a thermometer into this room and tonight when Daddy has his night sweats, I am going to take his temperature."

"Jill, he'll never let you. You're making too much of this, too much of a fuss."

She huffed and puffed as she tucked the sheets into the bed.

My father entered the room and looked somewhat guilty when he saw what was going on.

"Daddy, those night sweats you're having are not right. We've got to do something about them," I said.

"I'm going to take your temperature tonight. Is that okay by you?"

"I'm all right, Jill," he said. "I don't want to be any bother."

"You're here now and somebody's got to take care of you."

I gave my mother a mutinous look and left the room. I was tired and alone in the house with five children. One housekeeper came in each day, and the governess had taken ill herself. After the housekeeper left at five o'clock I was faced with the prospect of bathing Jason and Valentine, preparing a meal for all the children and my parents, carrying trays to the governess, and now I was going to get up to take Daddy's temperature. All this and nine months pregnant.

What would happen when the baby finally arrived, I did not know. Charlie was not due home for several weeks. My brother-in-law, Dempsy, arrived each morning to drive Suzanne and Paul to school, leaving me to drive the other three. They attended schools in all directions of the compass. I made myself a note to call an employment agency the next day for additional help before the house, which I already called the *Titanic*, listed any more to port.

I made myself another note to take my father to see Ray Weston, our family doctor, the next day. I was furious with my mother for bringing Daddy along in this condition without consulting a doctor.

I sank gratefully into a warm bath and had just begun to relax when my mother ran into the room in tears. She was literally wringing her hands.

"Jill, you've got to do something. Daddy's in terrible pain. Terrible pain. Do something. Get a doctor. I don't care if it costs all the money in the world. You've got to do something."

From my vantage in the tub, belly bulging, I was not in the best position to do something. But I hauled myself up, reminding myself to be careful not to slip and run the risk of injuring the baby.

"All right, I'm coming. Go back to Daddy. I'll be right there."

I pulled on a robe, telephoned Ray Weston, and went in to my father. It was true. He was in agony. His intestines were in knots. He was white, trembling in pain.

Ray arrived, gave him a sedative, and medication for pain. He told us we had to take Daddy to the hospital for tests the following day.

Their vacation was shorter than anticipated. A large tumor was discovered in my father's intestines; surgery was imperative. I was advised that for this particular surgery the best man for the job was a Harley Street physician in London. I drove my parents back to the airport after only a week. An ambulance rushed Daddy immediately upon his arrival to the hospital.

Two weeks later Zuleika was born.

19
Zuleika

1971

I sat on a hard but not uncomfortable hospital bed when Dr. Culiner arrived with a cheery, "Where's my girl?" as he walked into the room.

"Here I am," I said. "The pains are coming quite close together."

He came to the bed and rubbed my back, then smilingly said, "You're an old hand at this. It won't be any trouble. Want to play some gin rummy?"

"Sure."

Zuleika was born simply and quite swiftly. On her arrival, Dr. Culiner said, "She's got a lovely body. It's a girl."

I said, "You've got to be kidding."

He went into the corridor and told Charlie, "You've got a daughter."

"You're joking!" said Charlie.

Neither of us could quite believe I had given birth to a girl. But I had, and we named her Zuleika Jill Bronson. My first and only natural daughter.

Charlie and I named our daughter after a favorite novel

of mine, *Zuleika Dobson*, by Sir Max Beerbohm, of the famed Beerbohm-Tree theatrical family. I liked the similar sound— Zuleika Bronson, Zuleika Dobson, the wicked Edwardian scamp.

Charlie telephoned the children, who gathered in the kitchen of our Bel Air home awaiting the news. When I last saw them they were sitting gravely together in the entryway watching my departure. Ten concerned eyes followed me out the door.

When Charlie told them it was a girl, he said a big cheer went up, the loudest from Suzanne, who had announced the previous day, "If any more boys join this family, I'm leaving."

She was delighted to have a little sister. The boys were excited about the arrival of this child through whom flowed a part of all their blood, excepting Jason's. They had speculated on which sibling she would resemble—Tony's hair? Suzanne's eyes? Valentine's height? Paul's smile?

Jason had asked, "What will she have like me?"

I told him, "You will be the baby's big brother. The baby will love you, as I do."

Then, "Will you love the baby more than me?" to which I replied, as I did to all the children in turn, "You've got to remember I've loved you so much longer, so many years of love. It has to be more."

The night before I brought Zuleika home Jason had gone to Gigi, the nurse who had been governess to the boys and who would become Zuleika's nanny, and asked if he could climb into the white crib with its little lamb on the headboard.

Gigi, an Algerian of great sensitivity and intelligence, lifted Jason gently in her arms and deposited him in the crib as if he were a baby.

She later told me Jason, in his pajamas and fresh from his bath, curled up and lay looking around the room for some time before he asked her to lift him out again.

The next day I arrived carrying my precious bundle. The children trooped after me into the sitting room where I sank down on the couch where they clustered around to see their baby.

Zuleika awoke and opened her eyes. It was time for a bottle and I had one ready. The children watched her suckle.

"Can I try it, Mom?" Jason asked.

"Well, not this one, Jason."

But his face was so full of longing, I said, "Would you like to see what it's like to have a bottle? To see if you can remember?"

He said he would, so we all convened upstairs in the master bedroom where Gigi prepared a warm bottle of milk with a nipple. I put the baby in the small basket crib. Then, sitting down, I took Jason in my arms, wrapped a shawl around him like a swaddling and gave him the bottle.

The other children watched closely. Jason took a few sips, looking up at me almost as he had done as an infant.

"Yuck!" he said, and got up.

"Would anyone else like to try while I'm here?" I asked.

They all did, one by one. I cradled each child in turn and got the same "Yuck!" from each.

Next they sat cross-legged on the floor in a circle and each in turn held Zuleika in his arms to experience the miracle of life. Thereafter I retrieved my infant and put her to bed.

The children seemed satisfied by their foray into babyhood. None of them ever asked to have a bottle again.

I was a primitive mother; I kept the infant close to me at all times for the first few weeks of her life. I carried her around the house balanced over one shoulder doing my normal, everyday chores. And when I tired I simply lay on my back on the four-poster bed with the baby contentedly sleeping on my chest. It was during those private moments that the molecular structure of our bodies ebbed and flowed, the chemical bonding of parent and child. It was this confluence of energy, the primordial aura that surrounds mother and child, that had been missing in Jason's life after those first few heartbeats. It did not occur to me as I listened to the cadence of my infant daughter's breath that only Jason of my own four children had not had the chemical nourishment of this flesh-of-my-flesh bonding.

Zuleika was a round-faced, chubby little baby with a personality totally different from the boys'. She was definitely a little female. I loved her so much that one name never sufficed. Soon I began calling her by a string of nicknames, the first being Bun Face because of her full cheeks, Bubba because she was my Bubba. And then as she got older Tutti, then Tutu, then Bonnie Bun Face and Zulu.

The little girl agreeably responded to all the names. As she grew older I left her brief notes, addressing them to Miss Zuleika Bonnie Bun Face Bonwinkle Bronson, ending the message with two happy faces side-by-side. I had never before derived so much pleasure from the pure love I was experiencing. And, oh, what bliss it was to share this with her father, who loved her in an equally besotted way.

To have a child with a mother and a father under the same roof was a luxury for me. I had someone with whom to share and enjoy the daily occurrences involving Zuleika. Each daybreak was like Christmas morning. Charlie and I would awaken and look at each other smiling at the thought that we would soon see our beloved daughter. We raced each other out of bed to be first into the nursery to catch Zuleika's good-morning smile. Then we'd pick her up and bring her into our bedroom.

Charlie reserved a drawer in his desk especially for Zuleika. It was full of her things, funny bits and pieces that she and her father had placed there over the years. It was just the right height for a little girl. Her treasures included games, crayons, paper airplanes, small books, glass marbles. After breakfast Charlie often took Zuleika into the billiard room to stand her on the table where she ran around on the green baize, rolling the brightly colored billiard balls into the pockets. This bit of fun continued until she grew too tall and could no longer stand erect beneath the three hanging lights that illuminated the table.

I played records, then picked her up in my arms to dance around the room. She loved that.

When Zuleika was old enough to climb from her crib, she would awake in the middle of the night, swing herself down to the floor, bringing with her a favorite pillow and bottle. Then she would run as fast as her chubby legs would carry her down a long, dark corridor to the master bedroom where she would fling open the door with a bang and hesitate for an instant. Then we would hear *thump, thump, thump, thump, thump,* as she ran full-tilt boogie across the room, up over the foot of the bed to crawl under the covers between us.

I would wrap my arms around her little body and we would cuddle spoon fashion.

After a while Charlie would say, "She's asleep now, Jill, you'd better put her back in the crib."

Reluctantly, I would carry the warm, sleeping child into the nursery to her crib, place Dodo, a favorite doll, beside her and draw the covers over her, all the while inhaling the essence of her skin, her hair, her sweet breath, and the scent of the bedclothes. Often, rather than return to bed, I sat in the nursery rocking chair, and with the light of the moon blending with the dim nightlight, I would gaze at the baby while rocking quietly. I was not a new mother. I knew how fleeting and precious these moments were.

I somehow knew, too, that Zuleika would be my last baby, and I wasn't going to miss a moment of it.

We never left her as those first four years flew by. Zuleika accompanied us like a little gypsy on all of our travels. She was on the move so much during the first six years of her life the only consistent piece of furniture to which she clung was a collapsible crib that we took along.

She was a solemn-eyed, thoughtful little girl. For the first three years of her life she walked on her toes for the sheer joy of it. She loved running. She loved laughter and to be told stories.

Zuleika loved horses from her earliest years. The first time she encountered a horse on location in Almería, Spain, she studied it for a while and then went down on all fours and began eating grass. Frederick Ireland no doubt chuckled approvingly in the great beyond. As I'm sure did her great-grandfather William Eborn, my mother's father, who had been a mounted policeman.

Zuleika, the only Bronson-Ireland child in the family, linked Suzanne, Paul, Tony, and Valentine. I alone worried during the many dinner conversations speculating on just whose eyes, whose nose, whose chin Zuleika had inherited, and whether her hair would stay the same color as Paul's. Jason listened silently to the discourses of family resemblances. Charlie's family visited and conversations would be held about the distinctive Slavic family "look."

I once tried to bring Jason into it.

"Well, Jason, you've got my chin; the same cleft. You've got Paul's off-the-wall humor."

But there wasn't much Jason could say, and often my heart went out to him.

Despite my efforts to change the flow of those genetic conversations, they went on and on. Jason was so much a part of the family no one stopped to think he might be concerned by his natural exclusion.

20
Lifeline

"Zuleika," I said, "don't cry."

I was holding the little girl's hot hand in mine while smoothing her hair back from her damp brow. My daughter's gray eyes were filled with tears.

"Don't go, Mama."

"Baby, I must. I won't be long. I don't cry when you go to play with Tiffany, do I?"

Zuleika gazed at me wisely.

"But, Mama, I'm just a little girl. You are my lifeline."

21

Zip-A-Dee-Doo-Dah

1974

My mother and father were visiting us in Vermont, as was my small niece, Lindsay Ireland, my brother John's daughter. It was August and Zuleika, three, and Lindsay, five, had just celebrated their birthdays (four days apart) watched by their doting grandparents.

My father spent a great deal of time with the two little girls rambling in the woods. The songs of that summer were "Zip-A-Dee-Doo-Dah" and "Horsey Keep Your Tail Up." I can still see my father emerging from the woods at the back of the house into the clearing at the top of the hill some quarter of a mile away from where I sat in the breezeway.

He held each of them by the hand and the three of them were skipping along singing:

Zip-a-dee-doo-dah
Zip-a-dee-ay
My, oh, my, what a wonderful day!
Plenty of sunshine headin' my way.

By the time they reached the bottom of the hill I could hear the familiar refrain of "Horsey keep your tail up and keep the sun out of my eyes."

My father loved to sing and the children loved to join in with him. To them, who had not heard these songs before, my father was a miracle, a wealth of new ditties.

I would take the family for drives through the beautiful Vermont countryside in the long, dark-green station wagon. Daddy sat beside me in the front seat while Valentine, Jason, Zuleika, and Lindsay sat in the flat bed singing.

One day after dinner, as dusk approached, I decided it would be nice to drive my parents to see a particularly lovely nearby view. Paul and Charlie, Tony and Jason declined in favor of a ride on their motorbikes. I pulled on my large, brave pink hat I often wore while driving in those days and took off with Mother in the front seat beside me and Daddy in the back with Zuleika and Lindsay, who was singing "Zip-A-Dee-Doo-Dah" accurately and in tune.

We encountered Val on his bike, which he propped against a tree. He climbed in with us. It was growing dark. I told Val where we were going and he said he knew a shortcut. I believed him and we were soon lost.

On the darkening, tree-lined dirt roads we drove around and around identical byways. There were no houses, streetlights, or landmarks. Just more dirt roads and trees. There was no moon. It became black.

The strains of "Zip-A-Dee-Doo-Dah" had long since died away.

Valentine was navigating.

"To the left, Mom. To the right, Mom. That tree looks familiar, Mom," said the nine-year-old Val.

"Val, we're lost and I'm running out of gasoline. I'm not taking any more direction from you," I said.

I navigated a narrow lane leading toward a dimly lit dwelling. And suddenly, *bump*. All four wheels spun in the air beneath us. I had driven over a small hummock off to the side of the road. We were stuck and slightly airborne.

My father walked to the back of the large eight-seater vehicle, which weighed more than a ton, and strained to lift it off of the hummock. Mother remained in her seat, calmly confident he could do it.

I thought about his abdominal surgery in the not so distant past.

"For crying out loud, Daddy. Don't do that! You'll strain yourself."

Then out of the gloom and through bushes came four sinister-looking men.

"Could I use your telephone?" I asked.

I called Charlie from the house.

"I'm lost," I told my husband. "How do I get home?"

"Where are you?" he asked.

"I don't know. I'm lost."

"Then how can I tell you how to get home? Ask somebody where you are."

The woman of the house took the telephone and gave Charlie our location. Afterward Charlie said, "Get back on the road, go a half mile, turn left, and I think you'll know where you are. You're not really far from home. You're just confused."

"I can't," I said.

"Why not?"

"I've got the car stuck on a bump," I explained. "Daddy's trying to lift it off."

"Good Lord," Charlie groaned. "Can't somebody else help you? See what you can do and call me if you need me again."

Outside I discovered that with the help of the men the car was now ready to go, and we drove home.

Back in 1973, two days before my parents were due to return Lindsay to her parents in Canada, Daddy pounded his chest several times and began to do calisthenics, touching his toes, doing side stretches.

"This indigestion isn't getting any better," he said. "I can't seem to shift it with exercise."

His indigestion, however, did not prevent him from eating a hearty dinner that night; so I thought all was well. After dinner Daddy and I went into the attic to fetch a suitcase for my parents' trip. To reach the bag it was necessary to move several heavy steamer trunks and hard, old-fashioned suitcases. A particularly heavy case refused to budge for me.

My father said, "Let me do it."

I protested. "Daddy, it's too heavy. You can't do it yourself. Let me get one of the boys."

My father said matter-of-factly, "I'm strong, Jill. Look."

With one hand he grabbed the handle of the suitcase, packed as it was with ski boots, winter underwear, and sweaters. He raised and lowered the bag above his head four times in succession, a display of masculine dominance that both frightened and impressed me. It was true. He was strong.

I retrieved the suitcase and we returned downstairs. The next day Daddy left for Canada with my mother and Lindsay.

22

Toronto

1973

In Toronto two nights later Jack Ireland suffered a massive heart attack. My father was dying. I was devastated. I hadn't finished with him. I was not ready to let go. I rented a small two-seater airplane, put Zuleika under my arm, and flew to Toronto without a passport for either of us.

Once in Canada, I somehow convinced the airport officials to give me a special dispensation to stay in the country for two weeks.

John met us at the airport and we drove to see my father in the intensive-care unit. We were allowed inside one at a time. I found him sitting up bright-eyed, absolutely fascinated by the place. He was hooked to a fibrilator.

"It's really interesting in here, Jill," he told me. "You see all kinds of things."

His tone became confidential. Pointing to another patient, he whispered, "That one over there is going."

Indicating the blinking lights of the fibrilator, he said, "I'm going to be all right. My doctor told me people can be fine after a heart attack. I'll be left with just some scar tissue. I'll have to watch my diet, I suppose, but I'm going to be fine."

I said good-night, longing to tell him I loved him, but we just didn't do that in our family. My father hadn't kissed me since I was three years old. I could not bring myself to kiss him good-bye. Shyness got in the way. I was, however, able to fight for his life, as I discovered the following day when, because of overcrowding, he was moved out of ICU and into a private room.

I had registered at a small hotel nearby that soon became family headquarters. Lindsay and my mother stayed with me and Zuleika. Sandra, my delightfully wry sister-in-law—who is Scottish, attractive, willowy, highly intelligent, and a great chum—had given birth to her second daughter Courtenay two weeks earlier. Lindsay, whose nose was a little out of joint, was happy with the turn of events and delighted to see her cousin Zuleika again so soon. Sandra brought the baby for me to see and while I held the infant, Lindsay climbed on her mother's lap for a cuddle. The baby began to cry.

"Sandra, I think the baby's hungry," I said. "You better feed her."

Lindsay did not want to be put down and said, "You feed her, Aunt Jill."

I smiled and said, "I can't do that. Mommy must feed her."

Lindsay, with a five-year-old's exasperated know-it-all voice, came to me and said, "Of course, you can feed her. Just take that out and put it in her mouth." She pointed at my breast.

I explained only a mommy could do that for her baby, that only the mother gave milk; although other grown-up ladies had breasts, unless they recently had had a baby they did not have milk in them.

Displaced, Lindsay found her way onto her grandmother's lap.

The following day I arrived at the hospital to find my father, three days after a massive heart attack, out of bed and cranking, shaking, and readjusting his bedside table. I was angry. I had been told by Ray Weston that the majority of heart-attack victims suffered another attack within three days—if they were going to have another seizure. It was imperative my father stay in ICU, close to a fibrilator for at least three days. I got my father into bed and then called the hospital authorities.

I could not have my father moved back into ICU without his doctor's permission. I called the physician in charge of his case. He was on the golf course. I telephoned every country club in the Toronto area until I found the one to which he belonged.

"Put my father back into intensive care," I said.

The doctor's voice was slow, ponderous, and patronizing. "Mrs. Bronson," he said. "I think you're overreacting."

"Dr. Blank," I said. "I have both an emotional and financial investment in this. If anything happens to my father and he is not on a fibrilator, you will be surprised how I will overreact, as I'm sure you will when your bill is not paid."

Within the hour my father was back in ICU on a fibrilator. Just in time. He had three more heart attacks in rapid succession that night. The fibrilator saved him.

Daddy was forced to remain in Toronto for another six weeks.

On returning to England, to celebrate what he considered his complete recovery, my father dressed in a new sports jacket and was photographed by my mother's nephew, George, with a span of retired police horses. A horse nuzzled his hair. Daddy looked younger than his sixty-four years. He was a smiling, cheerful survivor.

Florence and Frederick Ireland would have approved.

23
Janet

1976

In 1976 I put together the first annual Zuleika Farm Horse Show, which was to become a popular, much anticipated event in the area. Many friends congregated at the farm to lend a hand. Among those who pitched in were Mark Farndale and teenage rider Stephanie Randolph, houseguest Jerry Nichols and Jane Ashley, my good friend and stable manager—all horse people and good hands around the barn.

The children joined in, too. Paul was eighteen, Jason fifteen, Valentine fourteen, and Zuleika six. The boys painted fences. Mark Farndale designed the course. They were festive, fun-filled days. My dogs, the aged Sara and Daisy, the half-coyote-half-German-shepherd mix, and crazy old Boris, the collie, ambled good-naturedly around, caught up in the "Hi-ho, Hi-ho" work atmosphere. Jerry, Mark, and I spent many nights putting together a program of classes for the competitors.

A few days before the show I received a telephone call from a woman I knew well from the horse-show circuit in California. Janet Berkoff. At the time I had no idea of the far-reaching and poisonous complications she would add to my life and my family's. She was a thirty-year-old woman who acted and looked sixteen. She wore her long, straight brown locks in a hairband like Alice in Wonderland. Janet affected a high, shrill, teenage voice and spoke in youthful idiom. She dressed in a style that these days would be called trendy. Her blue eyes on close inspection were surrounded by lines a touch too deep to be only laughter induced. But she did have a slender figure with small, high breasts that added to her general appearance of innocent youth.

She was the wife of a star tennis player on the professional circuit. Alex Berkoff loved his wife and indulged her passion for horses, cars, and fast living.

Janet's appearance, although pleasant, did not suggest a hot number.

She was a good horsewoman, a wealthy figure in a Rolls-Royce. There were rumors she was having an affair with one of the trainers, but that was none of my business.

I had known her only passingly. Her horses were stabled next to mine. Our tack boxes were situated side-by-side at the Los Angeles stables where we worked our horses. In spite of this, I was not surprised the day she telephoned from California to ask if she could participate in the Vermont show, saying she regarded young Stephanie Randolph as a protégé, her "little sister" as she called her. Janet felt left out and asked if she could come. I was surprised but happy to receive the extra company. The more the merrier was my motto in Vermont.

I drove the farm truck to meet her at the Lebanon airport. When she alit from the small commuter plane and walked toward me, I noticed a strangely pleading expression in her eyes, as if she were appealing to me for something. I didn't know Janet well enough to realize she was a deeply disturbed young woman.

I paid little attention as she played the life of the party in Vermont. She was adult in my presence, but when alone with the teenagers she got right down to their level and boogied with them, flirting outrageously with my young teenage sons. They were flattered. But fourteen-year-old Valentine, to whom she gave most of her attention initially, knew she was hitting on him; as he put it later with a wry grin, "I just wasn't ready for that."

But Jason, at fifteen, was. His masculinity was flattered by her advances.

On the night before the horse show Janet and fifteen-year-old Stephanie Randolph adjourned to the barn to braid the horses for the following day's festivities. Janet took along a bottle of wine. I was responsible for Stephanie, speaking to her mother in Los Angeles by phone every now and then, assuring her that Stephanie was being cared for properly. Four hours later, their horse braiding completed, Janet and Stephanie returned to the house. Stephanie was giggling and silly. She was obviously stoned.

When Janet came in, also giggling, she sat down with me for a woman-to-woman chat about the day's events. I was tense and hostile but nevertheless civil. Unaware of my disposition, Janet soon asked if it would be all right when we returned to California if Jason and Valentine came to the home of a Malibu neighbor to learn how to work the soundboard in her friend's studio.

"Valentine will love it, being a musician," said Janet, slightly slurring her words. "And Jason is really interested."

I held her in a cold stare and said coolly, "No, I don't think I'd like that, Janet."

"Oh," she said, startled, her blue eyes opening wide. "Why not?"

"Because, Janet, from my observation, I don't think you're a good role model and an example for teenagers."

Janet flushed. "Why are you saying that?"

"Look at Stephanie. Until you arrived she was behaving normally. Now she's obviously drunk or worse. I feel responsible to her parents, Janet. They trust my judgment."

"Well, you're wrong," said Janet. She flounced off to her room.

The next day she seemed to have forgotten our exchange. But Jason was sticking to Janet like glue. I told him and Valentine that I did not want them to accept Janet's invitation to her home when we returned to California. I was accustomed to being obeyed and put the matter to rest.

For the remainder of our stay in Vermont I was preoccupied with the show and other duties involved in the horse business. The next few days passed uneasily for me. I kept my eyes on the teenagers when they were around Janet. I suspected that what she handed out to them was more than candy. Coincidentally, my wine cellar depleted rapidly. It became apparent to me Janet had a great propensity for alcohol. It was with relief that I saw her depart.

I was curious why she had pursued my friendship in the first place, flying all the way from California to be part of what, after all, was little more than a small country show.

24

The Beginning

Kier lolled on the big bed at Janet Berkoff's Malibu home. He was smoking a joint. He luxuriated in having the time and attention of this brown-haired older woman whose eyes sparkled with as much mischief as his own.

Janet kept the vodka poured and provided a plentiful supply of high-quality cocaine. The white powder was arrayed in a series of pale lines on a marble-topped bedside table. She danced provocatively as she discussed the ladies-only party planned for the next day. She wore brief white tennis shorts and a clinging T-shirt. She was braless; her nipples strained against the much-washed cotton singlet.

Kier flicked the dials on the silent TV screen. Janet plopped herself down on the bed beside him.

"You want another drink, you little devil?" she asked coquettishly.

Janet reached over the table, suggestively thrusting her buttocks high in the air as she reached for the button that would dim the lights. Then she turned to Kier. "Don't you think it's time to go home, you little rascal?" she asked in her little-girl voice.

Kier took a long toke on the joint. Narrowing his eyes against the pungent smoke, he held the inhalation of weed in his lungs as long as he could. With one hand he reached out to the breasts that were offered for his eyes.

As Janet bent to kiss him, Kier felt strange stirrings of familiarity. He closed his eyes against the sight of the cloud of dark hair framing her face. He sank into a warm oblivious ecstasy, a place where all anxiety ceased to exist. The cavities within his body expanded and fit together. He was suddenly invulnerable to the insecurities and fears of Jason's world.

25

Busted

1976

It wasn't until the family returned to our Bel Air home from Vermont that I noticed a marked change in Jason's behavior. Some days he would disappear for hours without explanation. He was frequently late or absent from the dinner table. Jason had never previously been late to dinner without calling first or having a very good excuse. That was the way it was in our house.

The climax came the last day of October when at six o'clock Charlie was seated at the head of the English dining table, myself on his left and six children, who had washed their hands, seated along the sides. Each child had a rolled napkin pushed through a sterling silver holder bearing his or her engraved name. Guests were given a napkin and napkin ring with the engraved initial *B*.

My mother and father were visiting from England.

Charlie asked the boys, "Does anyone know where Jason is?"

No one did.

I had a strange, disquieting sense of uneasiness. This was not like Jason. I excused myself and called his friend Cory, whose sister Karen answered.

"Jason's not here, Jill. But I'll leave a message for Cory when he comes in. I think they're together."

I returned to the table. "Karen thinks Jason's with Cory."

"It figures," said Charlie. "Let's start dinner."

We all expected Jason to come bowling in while we were at table. But this did not happen. I spent the evening with Mummy and Daddy talking, reminiscing, and helping them wrap a few Christmas gifts they were leaving behind for the family on their return to England.

My mother picked up my concern. At one point she looked at the clock and said, "Where is that boy? He's so naughty worrying everyone this way."

At about eight-thirty the telephone rang. It was Jason.

"I'm at Cory's and I'm staying overnight if that's okay," he said.

"Jason," I said, "you missed dinner and you didn't call. I was very concerned."

"Sorry, Mom. Do you mind if I stay with Cory?"

"No. It's okay. I'll see you tomorrow."

"He's with Cory," I told my mother and father, to their visible relief. I told Charlie the same. "He's staying overnight."

"What about his homework?" Charlie asked.

"He said he and Cory will do it together."

"Huh," a disbelieving Charlie grunted.

I put Zuleika to bed, telling her, "It's okay, Jason's with Cory."

When I told Valentine, did I see a flicker of disbelief in his eyes? Or was it my imagination?

The next day passed with no sign of Jason. But I withheld this fact from my parents, who were unaware of the boys' comings and goings.

Charlie called Cory in the evening.

Cory said, "Jason's asleep."

"Wake him up, Cory."

Cory returned to the phone with another story. "I mean, he went out for something and he'll be right back."

"Cory, when Jason comes back, you tell him to come home right away or he'll be in big trouble."

By now the whole family was trembling under the rumble of Charlie's impending wrath.

I questioned Valentine. "What's he playing at, Val?"

"I don't know, Mom," the fourteen-year-old Valentine said miserably.

At eleven o'clock I received a call from Jason.

"Jason, what are you doing? You're not at Cory's."

"Yes, I am. And I want to spend the weekend here if it's okay with you."

"No, it is not okay. You must come home right away. Charlie is really angry."

"Sorry, Mom. I just need some time to myself."

"What do you mean, time to yourself?" I was exasperated.

"I have a lot of things to work out."

I became impatient. "What do you mean you've got a lot of things to work out? And why do you think you can work them out at Cory's instead of here?"

I had him at the end of the telephone line and wished I could reel him in.

"I forbid you, Jason. Have Cory or his mother drive you home immediately."

"I'm sorry, Mom, I need time to myself. I'm all right. Don't worry about me. Okay? I'm going now, all right? Good-bye, good-bye."

My God, the boy hung up. I was staring at the receiver as if it were a foreign object.

I punched out Cory's number, but it was busy and remained busy for the next hour.

"Charlie, what do you think he's doing?" I asked.

"Don't know, Jill. You know he and Cory are probably up to no good."

I drove to Cory's house two or three miles away.

Surprise! The place was empty except for Cory's grandmother, who was rather deaf and didn't know where the boys were.

Jason and Cory were pulling one of their stunts. I supposed Jason wanted to stay out later than his curfew. I remembered when Paul was the same age. His friend Jeff Howe would spend the night and I would visit the two fifteen-year-olds to bid them good-night. I can picture them now, Jeff in a sleeping bag on the floor at nine-thirty in the evening. Thereafter they would sneak out, hop on their bikes to go out to rock and roll—for crying out loud, whatever that was.

"Good-night, boys," I'd say.

"Good-night, Mom," Paul would answer, echoed cheekily by Jeff in his rasping, breaking voice.

"Sleep well," I would say innocently.

"Oh, we will," they'd chorus.

I'd no sooner close the door when they were out the window and on their bikes. When he was older, Valentine would do the same thing, feigning exhaustion at about nine o'clock, locking his door behind him.

The boys' wing was on the ground floor, so obviously out the window went Valentine. Except by now Mother was more experienced. One night I peeked through the keyhole in Valentine's room. His lair was strangely empty. So I went through Paul's room, the door of which was unlocked, through the adjoining bathroom, and lay down on Val's bed to wait. And wait I did, until one o'clock in the morning.

When my young night prowler returned through the window the room was dark and Valentine was obviously glad to be home. He sat with his back to me on the bed and with a sigh began to remove his sneakers.

It was then that the heavy hand of the law descended with a thump on his shoulder.

"Gotcha!" I said in a loud voice. "Gotcha!"

Valentine to this day remembers the shock.

"Oh, God, Mom. You scared the life out of me."

Because it was Val and because it was me, we both collapsed into laughter.

"Don't you ever do it again, Valentine," I said.

And because it was Valentine, he did not. Or at least he was never caught. He had gone to a forbidden late-night movie with a friend.

Although I was angry with Jason, it was not unusual for him to spend the night with Cory, and as I had heard all too often, boys will be boys.

This prolonged disappearance of Jason, however, was another and far more serious matter. Determined to find my son, I visited the homes of his usual friends and acquaintances. I telephoned others. None of them had seen or heard from him.

On the fourth day of Jason's disappearance, Cory came to our home and sat down with Charlie and me in our large, wood-beamed study. He said he felt guilty because he knew where Jason was.

"He's down at the beach with Janet Berkoff," Cory said, his head down.

His eyes began to fill with tears. "I feel bad because you've been so good to me, Charlie. This family has been good to me and I know how worried you are."

"Cory, please go and tell him to come home," I pleaded.

"I'll do it," he said. "I've been there before and I told him to come home. I told Jason he was acting like an absolute horse's ass. But he wouldn't come. I'll try again and I'll tell him you know where he is."

Late that evening Jason came home. Alex Berkoff was scheduled to return home from an overseas tennis tournament the next day, so I suppose Jason would have come dragging home anyway. When he did arrive, Jason had his tail between his legs.

I flung my arms around him. "I'm so glad you're home, darling."

Charlie stood quietly looking at him.

"It'll never happen again," Jason said. "But she loves me, Mom. And I'm in love with her."

Charlie and I looked at each other helplessly.

"But it's no good," Jason said. "Her husband's home now. It will be all over."

My sixteen-year-old Lothario retired to his room. Charlie and I naïvely thought that would be the end of that. But of course it wasn't. Janet was having too much fun with her little man, her toy boy. She continued her affair with my son, unbeknownst to us, and Jason's behavior became more and more erratic.

For his sixteenth birthday we gave Jason a black Jeep. Janet gave him a large bag of cocaine, which he hid in the basement, and a bag of marijuana, which he cached in Valentine's room, knowing we'd never look there.

Clearly, the situation was out of hand, but Charlie and I were in the dark about all this. Valentine knew. Cory knew. It was just another case of teenagers banding together. Nobody told.

I had never known such misery. Jason began going out at night and coming home late. I waited up for him. One night I was standing at the top of the staircase anxious and cold. I pulled my robe tightly around my shoulders. It was two o'clock in the morning. I heard the grandfather clock, which stood in our dining room, striking its mournful *bong, bong.* I looked out a window down to the front steps leading from the driveway and saw Jason making his way to the door in the early morning gloom.

I ran quickly down to open the door. "My God, Jason, I've been so worried. Where were you?"

My son stared at me with the expression of a trapped

animal at bay. "I wish you wouldn't worry, Mother. I've told you before. Don't worry about me."

His eyes were bloodshot and distended. He turned and walked away to his room, leaving the scent of alcohol. He had spent the evening with Janet. I knew because I had had him followed.

Eventually, I became so incensed by the midnight phone calls, the hang-ups when I answered, and Jason's unhappiness and confusion that I hired a private detective to have Janet followed. I also had Jason's telephone bugged, collecting masses of calls from all kinds of people. I learned more about friends, strangers, and acquaintances than I ever wanted to know. But eventually I got the material that would damn Janet Berkoff.

Her girlish conversations with Jason customarily began, "Hi, you little devil. How're you doin'?" and go on in a manipulative way, using her thirty-year-old wiles and neuroses to ensnare, charm, and corrupt my sixteen-year-old son.

During all this I enlisted the help and support of my young secretary, herself no more than twenty-five. She got caught up in the saga of Jason and his ongoing romance with Janet, and she fell in love with him herself. They began an affair, I learned to my horror through the bugged telephone line.

I had to listen to my own secretary discussing how she and Jason had such a good time the previous weekend, drinking champagne and snorting cocaine. Naturally, I confronted the girl and fired her, whereupon she broke down in tears, telling me she was passionately in love with Jason and pleading that I not let her go. She asked if, in the event she must leave, she could continue to see Jason.

I couldn't believe it. The situation was like "The Gong Show," but I couldn't gong any of the characters.

It was several weeks before I collected enough damning information to confront Janet. I searched my conscience carefully before deciding to act. I had to determine whether I wanted to hurt Janet or simply stop her from seeing my son. I was tempted to give all the information directly to Alex. Surely it would end their marriage and hurt Alex as much as it hurt her. My decision was to send my private investigator to a hotel where she was staying for a horse show in which she and I were both competing.

I was appalled to learn that Janet was staying with young Stephanie Randolph, whose trusting mother thought Janet provided a "big sister" image. I called Stephanie's mother and told her what I had discovered about Janet and Jason. But Mrs. Randolph obviously thought I was unbalanced. In any event, she continued to allow her daughter to spend much of her time with Janet.

So Stephanie was present in the hotel room when Janet was busted by my private detective and a member of the police vice squad. They told her quite simply that either she stop seeing Jason or all the information and tapes of phone conversations would be given to her husband.

I couldn't believe the scenario when the private investigator reported to me what took place.

Janet answered the door naked except for a towel. And when the investigator announced who he was, she asked, "Shall I come with you now?"

"That won't be necessary," he told Janet. "Why don't you put on a robe?" He asked Stephanie to leave the room before telling Janet about my knowledge of her contributing to the delinquency of a minor sexually and pushing drugs.

Janet promised she would never see Jason again.

That ended the seamy episode for Janet. I was satisfied, for the time being, with her promise. It was some small satisfaction that for the rest of her life Janet would know I held in my possession a safety deposit box filled with information and recordings of what had been going on between herself and a boy almost young enough to be her son.

Probably frightened by the threat to her marriage and her financial well-being, the loss of all those material things and status symbols that meant so much to her, Janet became pregnant as soon as possible. Almost a year later she gave birth to Alex's son.

Now, a decade later, I wonder if Janet, in terms of her own ten-year-old son, ever thinks back to the damage she did my son.

Somehow, once Janet was out of his life, I convinced myself Jason was back on the straight and narrow. If I had only known that nothing involving illicit drugs and alcohol is ever that simple.

In the meanwhile, life went on with the other children in an orderly fashion. Paul, Tony, Suzanne, and Valentine all graduated from high school and continued to live normal, healthy lives with the customary ups and downs common to young people. Zuleika grew up to be a happy little girl. Her main interest was horse shows. Katrina came to live with us at the age of fifteen and, after a period of mourning the death of her mother, also went into her life with an intelligent gusto and fortitude, which I admired.

It was only Jason who could not find his place in the world.

However, he did manage to get through high school and his graduation. How proud I look in the photograph taken of Jason in his robin's-egg-blue cap and gown, me with my arm protectively around his shoulders, clutching him as if I would never let go. I'd thought we had achieved something. I thought we had reached the end of a journey.

Instead, it was just the beginning. When Jason left school he spun out into the world with the abandon of a banshee.

26
Decision

1977

With methodical precision Jack laid out the items that he would pack into his suitcase, checking closely with the handwritten list he had made out earlier, in his distinctively elegant script:

Colostomy bags, belt, talcum, tape, cream.

Having put these medical necessities at the bottom of his bag, he then neatly folded his articles of clothing and added them along with his toiletries kit.

Overcome by an intense chest pain, Jack took a vial of amyl nitrite capsules from his breast pocket and popped two of them under his tongue. Quickly, the pain subsided. He completed his packing, closed the suitcase, and carried it to the front door. He was ready, looking forward to his trip. Nothing would spoil his visit with his daughter and grandchildren this time, he told himself.

Charlie, Zuleika, Valentine, and I waited at Los Angeles International Airport to meet my father, who was coming to vacation with us in Bel Air for three weeks. My mother and a close woman friend had gone to Paris on holiday. Daddy had just celebrated his seventieth birthday.

He bustled from the airport terminal excited to see two of his grandchildren. Charlie pulled up to the curb in my old blue Rolls-Royce with its JIB-1 license plate.

"Sit in the back with us, Grandpa," Zuleika cried.

So he did, squeezing between his granddaughter and Valentine. Charlie and I sat sedately in front.

On the way home, after all the usual *How are you's? How's grandma? How are the other children? How has the weather been?* the three in the back seat began a singsong.

My father was a great favorite with Valentine and his brothers. They loved his vast knowledge of rather ribald vaudeville songs.

"Sing 'The Three Old Ladies,' please, Grandpa," said fifteen-year-old Val.

I spun around on the pale-blue leather of the front seat, glaring at my father.

"Daddeeee," I said in a cautionary tone.

My father chose to ignore me and began:

Oh, dear, what a calamity
Three old maids stuck in the lavatory.
They were there from Monday to Saturday.
And nobody knew they were there.
The first one's name was Elizabeth Flicker;
She went to the lavatory with a dirty old vicar,
She thought she was quick, but the vicar was quicker . . .

"Daddy!" I cried. "I told you to . . ."

By that time Val was laughing uproariously. "Go on, Granddad, what is the next verse?" he egged his grandfather on.

"I can go pee-pee quickly," said Zuleika, not wanting to be left out.

"You see," I said. "Look what you've started."

"Go on, Grandpa," goaded Valentine. "Sing the verse about Elizabeth Humphrey who couldn't get her bum free."

At this I got up on my knees and said, "Daddy, you will not. That is enough!"

My father's brown eyes sparkled with amusement and I knew I sounded like my mother.

"We'd better listen to your mother or I'll get into trouble," said my father contritely.

Then I heard him whisper to Valentine, "I'll sing it for you later."

As the days of my father's vacation passed, Charlie, who took long walks with him, noticed Jack was short of breath and could walk only a few feet before stopping to pop an amyl nitrite pill in his mouth. He took those doses for granted but Charlie was appalled. All those pills could not have been good for him. My husband suggested we take my father to see Dr. Weston.

Much against his will, complaining and grumbling, he agreed to see Ray Weston.

Once more he had to hear Valentine ask, "If you're her father, Grandfather, how come she keeps giving you orders?"

Valentine had asked that question the first time when he was four and still found the situation puzzling.

With a characteristic shrug of his shoulders, my father got into the front seat of the Rolls and with a resigned, "Drive on," settled back, and let me take him to the doctor.

I waited two hours while my father underwent a battery of tests. When he returned to the waiting room and sat beside me, I saw concern in his eyes. His confidence had been shattered. At that moment Ray looked out through the receptionist's window.

"Jill, come into my office and bring Daddy with you."

I was warmed by Ray's reference to my father as *Daddy*. It made the forthcoming meeting seem somehow less ominous. I was wrong about that, though. We no sooner had entered Ray's office than he faced my father and said to him,

"John, I want to take you right to Cedars hospital. You must see a specialist. I don't believe you'll live much longer in the condition you're in. I think you need open-heart surgery."

"Don't say that, Ray. You'll frighten him."

"It's not a matter of frightening him. He's got to know the truth."

The whole exchange was turning quickly into a horror story.

The outcome of that visit was an angiogram at Cedars-Sinai Medical Center, which my father said was very uncomfortable. The cardiologist told my father he needed open-heart surgery. Five of his arteries were clogged. He marveled that Daddy had kept going. He needed immediate surgery.

My father had sworn never to go under the knife again, as he put it. "I didn't come over here for this, Jill," he said. "And anyway I have to talk to your mother."

That afternoon Charlie, Daddy, and I went out into the garden, followed by Sarah, the family dog. We sat in the shade of a large tree quietly looking out onto the gently rolling fairways of the Bel Air Country Club. My father sat a little slumped over, his large, capable hands resting on his knees. There still seemed to be quite a lot of youth left in him. And I'm sure there was hope still.

Suddenly, with an intake of breath, he raised his head and spoke words I would never forget: "I don't think I should have this surgery, Jill. I don't believe I need it. I have enough strength to carry me on as long as I'm supposed to go."

It was then that Charlie and I joined together, using all the powers of persuasion at our command, promising Daddy, as we had been promised, a better quality of life for him. More activity, sports again. We pressed home and finally persuaded him to allow surgeons to cut him one more time. He would permit them to perform open-heart surgery, a relatively new medical procedure at the time.

It is only now, having had experience myself with major

cancer surgery and the dread of possible recurrence, that I can understand the strength and determination of my father's resolve. The fear and resignation he must have felt as Charlie and I sat naïvely beside him with words of cheer and hope, watching his hands caress the old dog's head. We really didn't know what we were talking about. But Daddy did.

My mother was located in Paris and she flew immediately to Los Angeles. Charlie and I met her at the airport. Daddy stayed home with the boys.

Mother was nervous, apprehensive. "What do you mean open-heart surgery? What are they going to do? He said he didn't want more operations." My mother began to cry. "He's had so many. Jill, are you sure he has to?"

Then, pulling herself together, she said reassuringly to herself, "It's all right. I'll be all right in a minute."

She had been through this before. She watched my father submit to surgery of many types and descriptions, beginning at the age of sixty-four with intestinal problems. She watched while he suffered a massive heart attack and recovered. She stood by during three urgent intestinal surgeries, the last ending with a permanent colostomy. Yes, she knew her husband had had enough.

It was a quiet ride back to Udine Way where my father met my mother at the front door. Her personality immediately changed. She brightened and became full of cheery banter.

"Well, what have you got yourself into this time? I can't leave you alone for a minute, can I? Well, what's the matter? Are you jealous of all the attention I was getting in Paris?"

She put her arms around my father and they kissed.

"I'm tired," she said. "Let me go to my room. Let me see if I can remember. It's this way, isn't it?"

I was witnessing my mother taking up the gauntlet one more time. Daddy was obviously pleased to see her. And although he was smiling and making wry remarks, there was something about the set of his shoulders that was unlike him. Some of his cockiness had gone. No. All of his cockiness had gone. This was going to be much harder than I had anticipated.

But we did not have long to wait. The surgery was set for two days hence. So on a hot, balmy California evening we set out for the hospital, my mother, my father, my husband, and myself.

We all accompanied my father to his room. He was putting on a brave show, joking with the nurses, bragging about previous surgeries as he filled out the terrifying form that warned of all the horrendous things that *might* happen should this surgery be permitted. But of course, as anyone knows, it is just a formality. They have to tell you about all those things. It's not as if anything were really going to happen. Had we seen this form earlier, before the decision had been made, the situation might have been different. But now we were committed.

Charlie and I left the room while my father got into bed. I could see Daddy was already a favorite of the night nurse. He was evidently determined to be an incorrigible flirt to the last. Charlie and I bid him good-bye, saying, "We'll see you tomorrow."

I still wasn't able to utter the words, "I love you, Daddy." It wasn't our way. That was to come much later.

We waited in the car while my mother had a private moment with him.

"Oh, Charlie, I hope we're doing the right thing," I said.

Soon my mother joined us without a word. She was ashen. I could see she was trying not to cry. She held in her hands my father's personal possessions, putting his gold watch and other items into her handbag. They had been married more than forty years.

I turned to Mother. "How was he, Mummy? Was he all right when you left?"

My mother looked at me with pale, watery eyes. "Oh, he

cried a bit when I left. He always does. But he will be all right in a while."

"*He always does*" reminded me once again how many times my father had played this scene.

We drove home in silence. Open-heart surgery was still revolutionary, inspiring awe in the three occupants of the car. One could only wonder at the feelings of the man left alone in the tall, black-glass building of Cedars-Sinai Medical Center. After all, it was *his* chest they were going to open. It was *his* heart the surgeon would hold in his hand. It was *his* leg from which they would be taking the vein to replace the damaged arteries. Yes, one could only wonder what my father was thinking.

Left alone in the clean, impersonal hospital room, Jack felt diminished, less of a man. Would he ever feel the same? Be the same? Would he ever know the pleasures that required a strong-beating heart? He sat propped up uncomfortably on hard pillows. His blood had been drawn, the forms completed. The familiar dedignifying process of being prepared for surgery had begun. All he had to do now was wait. He listened to his heartbeat and marveled that in but a few hours a stranger wearing surgical gloves, his face covered by a mask, would open his chest cavity and reach deep inside. He had already been robbed of several of his faculties, his teeth, his spectacles, his hearing aid. They had all gone home with Doll. Would the surgeon tomorrow take what was left? His life?

The following day, after his surgery, I visited my father in the intensive-care unit. Only one visitor at a time, and only members of the immediate family. My mother had been the first to go in. Now it was my turn.

Daddy lay on his back, curtains drawn around him. He was heavily bandaged with a tube in his mouth.

I stood beside him and gently kissed him. Daddy's eyes fluttered open. He looked at me.

"Hello, Daddy," I said in a light voice. "How are you coming along?"

My father spoke the truth to me. "Oh, Jill. This is a terrible surgery. A terrible surgery."

As the days progressed my father got stronger and much of his cockiness seemed to return. He was through the worst of it and soon was back in his private room showing me the long white stockings they had put on his legs.

"Saucy, aren't they?" he asked. "All I need are garters. Want to take a walk with me, Jill? I am allowed to walk every day."

So I took my father along the corridors, admiring his strength and fortitude. Within days of his operation he was walking around with the twinkle back in his eye as he slowly forced his frame upright.

It seemed incredible that before two weeks had passed he was back home with us, lounging by the swimming pool with Mummy planning a fall vacation in England. We were all congratulating ourselves. I was jubilant. The right decision had been made. He was still a vital man with years of life ahead of him to enjoy the things he had always done. No more popping pills for him.

The time came for the family summer vacation in Vermont. Daddy and Mummy decided to come along for a couple of weeks before flying back to England. That way they could pick up three hours on their jet lag.

My father looked robust and debonaire, aided by the growth of a mustache during his ordeal. When we arrived in Vermont he spent most of his time sitting in a canoe on our largest pond, fishing for bass. Valentine joined him on those expeditions. They were quite successful anglers. The trouble was no one wanted to eat their prizes. Nevertheless they always brought their trophies home.

I had a TV tape camera and spent most of the two weeks photographing my parents. To my mother's delight and my father's annoyance, he is to be seen marching steadfastly toward the camera carrying a fishing pole and wearing one of my old straw hats. At my mother's insistence he would stop for a moment to smile condescendingly. Then he would head for the boat, walking out of frame with me, the earnest camerawoman, following him down the lane to the pond.

My mother was full of excitement and good humor. "Jack looks so much better, Jill," she said one day. "What a marvel. What a wonderful thing to be able to open somebody's chest and repair his heart."

They were happy days. Finally the time came for my parents to leave for England. I drove them to the Lebanon airport to catch the commuter plane to Boston.

Throughout his recuperation in Bel Air and during their stay in Vermont I never once heard my father complain of fatigue or pain. Instead, he kept up his steady teasing banter, jokes, and songs. He was popular in the boys' room at night. They went upstairs saying, "C'mon, Grandpa, you promised."

My father walked up the stairs, turning to us to say, "Stag. No women allowed."

The door closed. There would be a few moments then gales of hearty masculine laughter with pounding of boyish feet on the floor. Charlie would look at me and roll his eyes. We could imagine the pictures falling off the walls in the boys' room with Paul, Tony, Jason, and Valentine rolling around clutching their sides as father delved deeper into his scrapbook of jokes suitable only for teenage boys.

Charlie preferred to stay with the womenfolk. He, my mother, Zuleika, Suzanne, and I sat around in the breezeway drinking herb teas, resenting the refinement of our activity. Zuleika, particularly, I could tell, ached to sneak up the back stairs and listen at the door. Zuleika loved her grandpa. He knew just the right way to tease her.

The cool evenings were spent with my whole family playing hearty games of baseball. My mother and I called it rounders. My father umpired. Dorothy proved herself to be pretty good with the bat. And when she hit the ball there was a resounding chorus of "Run, Grandma. Run, Grandma" as my mother, her cotton skirt flapping at midcalf, ran as fast as she could in her new sneakers. My father, laughing, joined in, "Come on, Grandma, run."

As she neared second base, her legs wobbling, Jason shouted, "Slide, Grandma, slide!"

All too soon it was time to say good-bye to my parents at the airport, telling them the next week Zuleika was to enter her very first horse show.

"I'll write and tell you all about it," I said as Zuleika kissed them both good-bye.

My father left with such high expectations, he took his new fishing pole with him, carrying it over his shoulder. His new mustache had grown quite bushy and his hair long, as I liked it.

"God, Jack, you look like a character actor in a western," said Charlie.

"Yes, you do, Jack. You'll get a haircut when we get back," my mother said bossily.

"No," I protested. "Don't make him get a haircut. I love it long. He looks good, doesn't he, Charlie?"

"He looks good," the boys chorused. "Good-bye, Grandpa."

"Good-bye, Grandma."

"Slide, Grandma!" Jason hollered.

"Good-bye, Jack. Good-bye, Dorothy," said Charlie.

I hugged my mother. "Good-bye, Mummy."

"Good-bye, Jilly dear. Thanks for everything," she said.

I hugged my father. "Good-bye, Daddy."

"Good-bye, Jill. You've been a real brick through all of this. Hasn't she, Doll?" He motioned to my mother, who nodded, choking back tears.

These were the last coherent words my father would ever say to me.

27

Seaford, Sussex

1977

Jack sat in the sunhouse, warm and dozy in the September sun, happy he had built this small brick-and-glass house. Built it by himself, he had, he told himself in a congratulatory way.

He did all the work after his heart attack, when everyone said he wouldn't be able to do it. Shouldn't do it, because of his heart. But Jack had known he could mix the cement and carry the bricks from where they had been delivered in the road outside their bungalow. It had taken a few weeks, but it was done.

Now Jack and Dorothy used the little summer house most afternoons, basking in the watery English summer sun, the glass windows intensifying its rays.

They would sit together companionably reading or just chatting.

The wall behind him, as he sat in the deep garden chair, was hung with his paintings. He was planning another canvas depicting his daughter's house in California where he had just spent so much time. But that, he told himself, would be after the fall vacation he and Doll would take, a tour around the lovely English countryside. They would enjoy the colors of the autumn leaves, just the two of them, Jack mused.

Oh, he felt so much better after the open-heart surgery. His spirits soared. Now they would be able to walk through the country lanes, maybe even hike along the cliffs at the top of the Seven Sisters, the craggy heights that bordered the ocean close to Beachy Head and their home in Seaford.

How they had loved that walk when they first moved to Seaford. Jack felt a sadness as he remembered it had been out of the question for a long time now because of his heart condition. But with five new valves pumping blood through his body, Jack was full of renewed vigor. His body twitched, telling him to move, to exercise, the way it had in his young manhood. It was wonderful to feel so rejuvenated.

The scar that ran the length of his chest from his collarbone to his diaphragm, had already faded to a fine white line in only six weeks. He was a new man.

Jack glanced in the direction of the kitchen window. He saw his wife moving around, making lunch for them both. She would be calling him soon. It was about that time. Maybe he had time for a stroll before lunch. He began to rise from his comfortable garden chair.

A sudden sickening wave of light-headedness hit him. Jack sank down again. He had arisen too quickly. He would wait a second, then try again.

28
Green Ribbon

I was happily returning to the Vermont farm from Zuleika's very first equestrian competition, driving the truck pulling the horse trailer. Zuleika had ridden Turtle and we were coming home triumphantly clutching a bright green ribbon. The fact that every competitor in the class that day had been given the identical green ribbon did not daunt us. The blue ones would surely follow in good time.

Zuleika had been practicing most of the summer, sitting high and tall on the back of Turtle, who was not a horse to be trifled with. He was not a suitable mount for a little girl, but we led him around.

Turtle was braided this hot August day. Even in all the heat Zuleika properly wore her navy-blue school blazer and white shirt with a little red necktie and velvet helmet. She did not yet have a proper show hacking jacket, but the blazer looked just fine, at least for this class. She wore a brand-new pair of riding boots and breeches. It was a very excited little girl who was led into the ring on Turtle, his coat gleaming.

It was such a hot day that afterward I took off her warm

woolen jacket and we put our feet in a nearby stream and ate our lunch. Towering trees shaded the brook, filled with boulders large enough to hold a feast for one happy mother and seven-year-old victorious child clutching her first ribbon.

After lunch we got into our truck and wended triumphantly back to Zuleika Farm.

"Zip-a-dee doo-dah, zip-a-dee-ay. My, oh, my, what a wonderful day. Plenty of of sunshine . . ." sang my daughter.

Chiming in with the harmony as we drove up the tree-lined driveway, I waved the ribbon out the window at Charlie, who stood at the front of the house awaiting our arrival.

Zuleika and I scrambled out of the truck happily, dogs bounding out behind us. Zuleika ran to her father. "I've got a ribbon. I've got a ribbon!"

Surprisingly, Charlie did little more than say, "I see, baby. That's very nice."

I expected a more boisterous demonstration of paternal pride. Instead, Charlie looked at me and said, "Come inside, Jill. I've got to talk to you."

Once indoors and out of Zuleika's earshot, my husband said somberly, "Your mother's been calling all day from England."

A flutter of alarm deep inside my chest cavity forced me to study Charlie. His face was inscrutable.

Then his words: "Your father's had a stroke. Your mother wants you to call as soon as possible."

I sank onto the small couch facing the fireplace and grabbed the telephone.

My mother quickly confirmed the news, saying, "I'm not a wicked person, Jill. I'm not. But if I thought he would have to live this way . . ."

"Of course you're not wicked, Mummy. Tell me what happened."

"Well, your father was sitting in the sunhouse reading. It was a lovely day. When I called out to him to come for lunch, he didn't move. He just stayed there, sitting. After I put the meal on the table, I went into the garden and saw something had happened. He was sitting in his deck chair trying to get up but he couldn't.

"He was trying to move his leg. He couldn't speak or look at me. I realized something was terribly wrong. I called a neighbor and somehow we managed to get him into the bedroom. Dr. Bains came quickly and said Jack had suffered a stroke. They took him to hospital. Oh, Jill, I can't believe it. After all he's been through . . ."

As I listened, I felt as if I were slipping down a huge well of misery. The same slippery well my father had so painstakingly climbed, hooking his fingers over the top to haul himself up and out into the sunshine of "Zip-a-dee Doo-dah," when a huge hand unprized his fingers and pushed him back down the well.

"I'm coming over, Mummy," I said.

We said good-bye. The children all piled into the sitting room and sat around watching me. I was stunned. I could not believe the horrible news. Worse, the situation was out of my hands. There was nothing I could do. I began to cry.

"What's happened to Grandpa?" Zuleika asked. She was clutching Julie July, the doll she had adopted the year before, saying she had so many dolls she decided only one would be special.

I looked across at Charlie.

"I've got to go to England, Charlie," I said. "I've got to go. Do you understand?"

Charlie said he did.

29
Brighton

1977

I packed a small bag and the next day Paul, Zuleika, my oldest and youngest, and I drove a rented car to Boston where we caught a plane for England.

In London I was met by Charles Yates, a longtime friend. He drove us to Brighton where I took three adjoining bedrooms and a small sitting room at the Grand Hotel overlooking the sea. Mother joined us.

My mother was by now stoic, teary-eyed but stoic. Life was supposed to be going so well, yet she found herself the wife of a man with whom she could not communicate.

She told me that when my father regained consciousness he was unable to speak. It is curious to note, however, that when he recovered his senses Jack was singing "Waltzing Matilda" at the top of his lungs. The nurses, who did not know him, thought perhaps he wasn't an Englishman because when he spoke he made no sense. He had lost the use of his right arm and they feared he might be paralyzed in both legs.

He attempted to communicate by writing, almost convincing the nurses he was Egyptian because his penmanship bore more relationship to hieroglyphics than anything they had seen before.

He was, my mother now knew, suffering from aphasia. A blood clot in the left side of his brain had destroyed his powers of communication, the use of his right arm and leg.

"He hasn't tried to talk to me, Jill," my mother said. "All he does is look sadly up as if he doesn't know what hit him."

"Well, he probably doesn't," I said. "Has anyone told him he's had a stroke."

"I don't think so."

Dorothy Ireland had pulled herself together and was no longer the weepy woman I had spoken to on the telephone from Vermont. Before leaving the hotel for the hospital we ordered a small egg custard from room service, carried it carefully to the back seat of the hired car, and the four of us drove to the hospital.

On the way, out of nervousness, my mother and I bickered.

"Mummy, you're not holding the custard straight. It's going to spill."

She gave it to me rather briskly, and it did spill on my skirt.

"Now look what you've done; you've spilled it on me."

"No, I didn't. It was your fault."

Stupid bickering from two women terribly distressed about the same man.

We arrived at the hospital and walked through the stone corridors, bordered by walls painted institutional green, and located Daddy's ward. We were greeted by the matron, a friendly Englishwoman who did most of the patient caretaking. "He knows you're coming, Mrs. Ireland, but he doesn't know your daughter's here. We weren't sure she would be here today, and nobody wanted to overexcite Mr. Ireland. He's about the same as he was yesterday."

The large ward was attractive, a big room with lots of

light and windows looking out onto a blue sky. It was two rooms, basically, with four beds in each segment. My father was in the far room, his bed with its back to a wall. The four men in the first ward looked up as we entered, hoping we were visiting them. And then with either a smile or blank expression, they looked away and went back to their own thoughts. This was a room full of men without much hope.

As I entered, I heard a growling sound in tones that I understood to be my father's. My eyes traveled to him. He still had his California suntan and his dark eyes burned with intensity and life. He saw me and fastened his attention on my face with an almost superhuman life force. He gasped.

I walked quickly to his bed, followed by my mother, Paul, and Zuleika. My father gasped again and then broke into sobs. From his lips came unintelligible sounds. Not one word could be made out.

I quickly sat beside him, stroking his head and kissing his cheeks. I noticed that one hand was out of sight under the sheets, but his good left hand was still strong and suntanned. The corner of his mouth was just slightly turned down.

"Daddy, you're going to be all right," I said. "Do you hear me? You're going to be all right. Do you know what happened to you, Daddy?"

"Ah." He stopped for a moment and gave me a questioning glance. He trusted me. This was his daughter from America who had always made things right, who had always come to his rescue, the one who had flown in the private plane without a Canadian visa when he suffered his heart attack. The one who suggested heart surgery that was supposed to save his life. The one who perhaps was responsible for his predicament right now.

I said to him, "Do you know what's happened to you, Daddy? You've had a stroke."

I could see by his eyes that he understood. I proceeded to explain to him exactly what had happened and was rewarded with the light of comprehension in his eyes.

He made it known he wanted to see himself in a mirror. I took my compact from my purse and held the glass to his face. He inspected his mustache, moving his mouth from left to right. I realized he wanted to see the extent of the damage the stroke had wrought.

"What are you doing, Jack? Checking your mustache?" my mother asked.

"No. He wants to see how he looks. He remembers stroke victims with distorted faces. You're still a handsome devil, Daddy. You still look great. And your speech will come back if you work on it. You're going to be fine, really fine."

He seemed satisfied. Everything appeared to be in order. He returned the compact to me.

Zuleika was holding Julie July. Now she approached her grandfather. He had always teased her about the doll, taking it on his knee, holding its torso in one hand and making its head wobble, saying, "Oh, my poor granddaughter. Poor little Julie."

Zuleika, remembering this and attempting to help her grandfather, placed the doll on the bed beside him and said, "Julie has come to visit you, Grandpa."

My father looked at Zuleika, turned his head, and said gently, "Ah."

Zuleika had been told her grandfather could not speak and that we were all going to try to help him.

"Would you like to play squiggle?" she asked.

"Ah," said my father.

And that's just what they did for about three minutes. Zuleika made a squiggle and with his left hand my father tried to make it into a picture. Then he would make a wavering line and Zuleika made it into a picture.

It was the first time my father had tried to communicate. I was so very proud of the little girl and her intelligent efforts to help her grandfather.

Paul tried too. He took my father's hand in his and said

to him, "Grandpa, if you understand me, squeeze my hand once for yes and twice for no."

But this means of communication did not get them very far. My father was tiring physically. I fed him the egg custard.

The first visiting day was over and we returned exhausted to the hotel.

For two weeks each day was the same. Paul and I arose early, pulled on our running shorts, and tried to stay asleep, as we put it, while we ran four miles along the sea front. This was a possibility. One's body can still function while the brain is sleeping. Then we returned to the hotel, showered, changed, and picked up Zuleika and my mother to visit the hospital.

My father recovered rapidly after the first few days, amazing the hospital staff by swinging his legs over the bed and standing up. I put on his robe and then tucked his now paralyzed right hand into his pocket, thus making his affliction less obvious.

The nurses told me how independent they found him. Jack refused to let anyone help him bathe. He was determined to do as much for himself as he could. His speech was another matter. He didn't seem to understand that nobody could make sense of his *lo lo los*. The only words that came out clearly were those I had never heard him utter—"fucking hell."

The specialist at the hospital had cautioned us that his first words would probably be profanities. As it turned out, they were the only words he would ever say. So "fucking hell" became conversation to him. Whereas once he would say, "Oh, really," he would now say "fucking hell" in the same tones, which did have its amusing points, but hardly moved the conversation along.

During the time I watched my father's progress my mother and I met with a specialist. Ray Weston called from Los Angeles to say, "Don't give up on this man. He may be seventy, but there is a lot of life left in him. He's not an ordinary man. Don't give up on him."

I knew in England the tendency was to say that such cases had lived their three score years and ten, and this was the order of things. They would probably just gently let him die. Ray beseeched Daddy's doctors to give him a drug to shrink the tissue surrounding his brain immediately after the stroke, reducing the inflammation. He said if the drug were administered there would be minimum brain damage.

The specialist, however, refused, saying it was a controversial and unproved drug in England.

The same specialist looked at me and said in a rather highhanded manner, "I know you're from America and think you know everything . . ."

My mother interrupted immediately. "She's just a very worried daughter, doctor."

I was furious. I wanted to slap the man.

He said, "You must be philosophical. I lost my father to a stroke last year. These things happen."

I could see that any help for my father would have to come from himself.

That night my mother and I went to a restaurant while Paul baby-sat for Zuleika. We had dinner and a few glasses of wine. Over to the table came a man playing an accordion. My mother immediately brightened and began to sing, joining the accordionist with old favorites. I joined in.

My mother and I always had the ability to temper tragedy with a little humor and lightheartedness when we got too low. We *had* to. I noticed the same quality in Katrina when her mother died. She could cry for only so long, then she had to go out and play with Zuleika; I would hear her laughing in the garden. This night my mother and I drank a bottle of champagne and came rolling home to the hotel. We walked along the corridor to the suite in the Grand Hotel in Brighton, giggling like a pair of schoolgirls.

Fumbling, I placed the key in the door, opened it, and

found my ex-mother-in-law, my ex-brother-in-law and his daughter with Paul.

Entering in a most undignified way, I said, "Whoops! Let's go out and make this entrance again, Mother."

Which we did.

Paul had welcomed the visitors, who decided to await my return. Dorothy McCallum, an attractive auburn-haired woman with bright blue eyes, was in her late seventies. She had been prepared to be sympathetic, as indeed she was. It was nice to see her and my former brother-in-law, Ian.

Throughout the difficult stay in Brighton, Paul was a wonderful friend, ally, and number-one son. While at the hotel, my burly teenager put quite a dent in my reputation with the maids on our floor. He did not deign to use the corridors to enter my room, choosing instead to climb over the balconies and through my window, often wearing running shorts and sometimes pajamas. At least two maids and one room-service waiter were aware that a scantily clad, handsome lad entered my room through the window regularly. Many an eyebrow was raised.

After two weeks we returned to the United States, piling back into Charles Yates's car, waving to my mother who stood, a lonely figure, on one of those balconies, a small handkerchief fluttering in her hand as we pulled away. I felt as if I were deserting a sinking ship, but my home was in America. My husband and children awaited our return.

Paul, Zuleika, and I made our sad little voyage back to Vermont. I had a particularly heavy heart because I felt that if it hadn't been for the open-heart surgery, the stroke would have killed my father, or perhaps he wouldn't have suffered the stroke at all. At the same time, we still had hope he might regain his speech and the use of his arm.

In the following few years we would drag Daddy to every speech therapist and physiotherapist that London and California had to offer.

We were told the best chance for communication was

Daddy's ability to write with his left hand. At this news we plummeted into despair. There was no way any of us could understand anything he ever wrote. It appeared he would never communicate with us again. His attempts at miming were oblique and never to the point. For instance, one night he wanted to tell us he did not wish to eat dinner. Instead of simply patting his stomach, shaking his head, or covering his mouth, he went into an elaborate mime, tracing out a rectangle in the air accompanied by lots of gibberish and ending in frustrated tears. This was two years after his stroke. The rectangle he had inscribed we eventually understood was simply his place mat.

But these were early days and we still hoped. As the years passed, two years, four years, he still did not speak or write more than one coherent word at a time.

Daddy was a very different man from the one who had occupied our guest room before his heart surgery. At least on the outside he was. Inside, I was horrified to see my father looking out at me, lost and bewildered, still frustratedly attempting to reach us with words so clear and plain inside his head. But they came out of his mouth gibberish or *lo lo lo*.

I read literature by the yard concerning aphasia. The book most clearly describing my father's condition was written by a doctor in his forties. He had had a stroke and was taken to the hospital. He recovered consciousness but did not know what had happened. He tried to ask a nurse who, it appeared to him, was either deaf or did not speak English. She failed to understand his perfectly clear question. His wife had gone home, the nurse told him, and would return shortly. The young doctor reached for the telephone and dialed his home. When his wife answered, he asked what had happened and requested she bring his spectacles and pajamas when she returned.

His wife did not respond. She repeatedly told him everything would be all right, that she loved him and that she would return to the hospital immediately. He became frustrated and hung up.

In the book this same scenario is written from the wife's point of view. It was Kafkaesque to them both.

After her husband was hospitalized, she waited for him to regain consciousness. Finally, exhausted, she had driven home. When she answered the telephone she recognized her husband's voice. But she could not understand a word he spoke. She heard incoherent babbling, ending in shouting. She could think of nothing to say except to assure him everything would be all right.

As I read the book I'm afraid the pages were dampened many times with my tears as I thought about how it must have been for my father those first few days in the hospital when he, too, babbled urgent requests to his family and we replied how much we loved him and that everything would be all right.

But it was not all right, and never would be again.

Before leaving Brighton, I had written a long, detailed letter to my father, explaining carefully just what had happened to him. I reminded him of actress Patricia Neal who had suffered a similar stroke and had learned to speak again. I did not mention that Miss Neal was in her thirties at the time, and, unlike my father, did not suffer deafness.

My mother said Daddy reread the letter many times, then folded it up in his one good hand and put it away at the back of a drawer.

On his first poststroke visit to Udine Way in November of 1978 it was never more clear to me that inside his head Jack Ireland was the same man he had always been. After dinner the family left the two of us at the table. Everyone was exhausted from the constant Twenty Questions throughout the meal with my father playing master of ceremonies.

I looked into his eyes and to encourage him, I said, "I think it's wonderful, Daddy. You're walking again. You're doing so well."

Face to face we looked at each other. My father, peering deep into my eyes, slowly shook his head. I could see Daddy looking out. I could hear what he was saying in my mind:

"No, I'm not, Jill. It's not wonderful. I'm not doing so well. This is me in here. Don't patronize me. I am not a child."

I felt the words. I said to him, "Oh, Daddy, don't look at me like that. You'll make me cry. Let's have a drink."

"Lo lo lo," he said, reaching out with his good left arm for the half-full bottle of wine. He filled our glasses and we drank them down like greedy children with milk and cookies.

I would never agree that my father had gone. No matter what anyone told me, I would never accept the easy solution: that this man was no longer the same because he could not speak, or that he was in some way diminished mentally.

Despite being locked in the prison of his own head, the successful quintuple bypass heart surgery had strengthened him physically. He walked two or three miles every day around the UCLA campus, making his paralyzed leg sturdy. With the aid of a walking stick and with his paralyzed right arm tucked in his pocket, the casual observer would have seen a rather distinguished, white-haired older gentleman marching with determination and alacrity, taking his constitutional.

I worried something might happen, that he would be unable to explain to people who he was or where he came from. So I removed my old *Medic-Alert* medallion and had my name and allergic problems removed. In their place I had inscribed: *Jack Ireland, aphasia victim, cannot speak but understands everything*.

I added his telephone number in England and gave it to my father. And because it was a gift from me, he wore it proudly.

During that first poststroke visit, the family congregated for Charlie's birthday. I brought in a birthday cake ablaze with candles. No sooner did I appear in the darkened room than my father's voice rang out ahead of the others:

"Happy birthday to you. Happy birthday to you. Happy birthday, dear Charlie, happy birthday to you."

It was incredible. We understood every word he sang.

So astonished were we that no one else joined in. I know there were tears in my eyes.

Since that time, singing has been a major means of reestablishing a sense of continuity in our lives, a touch with past memories.

Sadly, however, Daddy can only sing old songs with no relevance to communicating thoughts or feelings.

Perhaps my father was just too old. Maybe help didn't arrive in time. It was difficult to get sufficient therapy in Sussex. A therapist visited him once a week, scarcely enough. My mother became Daddy's constant therapist. We continued to cling to every hope that we could bring my father back to what he was.

While my mother dealt with the hard facts on the home front, I searched my mind and battered my conscience with recriminations.

I asked myself how I could have been so sure in persuading him to have the heart bypass operation.

He had told me in his own distinctive voice, "I don't think I should have this operation, Jill."

Perhaps we should have let him go in the full stride of his manhood.

Oh, I had a pat answer for everything, interfering with fate. I could see now there are worse things than death . . . living death. Or was I wrong?

Ignorance is bliss and wisdom always comes too late it seems.

30
Cissie

1981

When Jason was eighteen he met a young Englishman, Nigel Webster, who invited my son to stay with his family in England. I thought it would be good for Jason to get away and stand on his own two feet, perhaps to find his own identity in a far-off land.

Jason worked as a bartender. He fell in love with England and he fell in love with Nigel's fifteen-year-old sister, Cissie. She was a long-legged uniformed schoolgirl, a cute, round, and bubbly little thing with soft brown hair and a tomboy quality. She spoke in a light but husky cockney accent. Jason had never seen or heard anything quite like her. The Websters liked Jason and encouraged the relationship.

As luck would have it, when the time came for Jason to return to the United States, Cissie's sister, Angela, was coming to Los Angeles to live with her husband. Cissie and Jason were ecstatic when her family allowed her to accompany her sister; the two young people would not be separated. The romance would continue. And this it did for a couple of years.

Jason rented a house in Venice and when Cissie turned sixteen, she moved in. They began buying furniture and putting up family photographs. They adopted a little black cat and they became a family.

I visited one day and was happily surprised to see what a comfortable and attractive nest they had made together. Cissie was the sort of cook that a nineteen-year-old young man could appreciate. She made wonderful bangers and mash on the gas stove in their little kitchen, and brewed large pots of British tea.

Then Jason got a job in a movie company that traveled to Mexico. Cissie had begun a fledgling modeling career and could not leave with my son because she was to be photographed the following week. Jason went to Guadalajara and began his job enthusiastically. After only two weeks he received a hysterical phone call from Cissie at two o'clock in the morning.

She told Jason she had been raped by the photographer who, by chance, was also a friend of Jason's. Jason went berserk. He insisted she join him immediately. But he could not contain the anguish and rage when he saw the bruises on her body. The impassioned nighttime conversations began to take their toll on Jason, what with movie work hours beginning at dawn. He reported to the set red-eyed, unshaven, and exhausted. He began drinking in the evenings. His inner turmoil and frustrated rage got the better of his always sensitive digestive system. He began vomiting blood.

It was clear Jason could not continue to work while in the throes of such torment. He loved Cissie. He called her his baby—and someone had raped her!

Jason left his job and with a tearful Cissie in tow returned to Los Angeles where Cissie was to meet with police officers investigating the case. But Jason had a darker purpose. He wanted to have words with Cissie's assailant. The photographer had left town. But the burden of the catastrophe was too brutal for the young people. Cissie telephoned her mother and Mrs. Webster insisted that she come home. Badly shaken and needing to be with her mother, Cissie left Jason, promising to write and return to him soon.

They never saw each other again.

Once more a malevolent star had cast a shadow on the light that should have shone protectively around Jason.

Perfectly capable of making enough trouble for himself, this time Jason was blind-sided.

31
Katrina

1982

In 1982 I became involved in the production of a movie based on a book I had bought with two partners two years previously. It was titled *The Evil That Men Do* and was to star Charlie. As associate producer, I was introduced to Hilary Holden, an Englishwoman who was the casting director. Hilary and I got along like a house afire. For two months we worked side by side, brown-bagging our lunches, discussing our lives and our daughters. Her daughter, Katrina, was fourteen. Zuleika was eleven.

Hilary was single and adored her only child. She lavished love and attention on Katrina and had sent her to ballet school for years. I met the child only twice when she floated into our offices after school. Katrina was a thicket of arms, legs, knees, elbows, hands, and feet. Her hair was long, dark, and wild. Her brown eyes were alive with mischief and fun.

I went to Mexico when production began. Hilary stayed in the home office. When I returned, filming completed, Hilary and I decided to open a production office. We had dinner and spent the evening planning, designing our office, and discussing books that might make good film properties. I was to speak to Hilary by telephone several times after this meeting, but I never saw her again. She died of a heart attack Friday the 13th, May 1982.

Charlie and I were awakened by the telephone. It was four-thirty in the morning. Charlie answered. Pancho Kohner, a producer and friend, was calling.

Pancho, himself divorced and living alone, did not know what to do. He telephoned us. "Hilary Holden is dead," he told Charlie.

"What is it, Charlie?" I wanted to know.

He turned to me. "Hilary's dead."

I didn't believe it. "Hilary? NO! Oh, my God, no."

I took the receiver from Charlie.

The sound of the crying child was heart rending. "Darling, this is Jill. I'm coming to get you. Do you hear me, Katrina? I'll be right there."

Oh, God, I wanted to scream in rage, to cry, but there wasn't time. There were other priorities. I had to get to Katrina.

Katrina had shared Hilary's bed that night to comfort her mother until she fell asleep. Hilary, who wore a pacemaker, suddenly awakened screaming and breathing strangely. Katrina gave her mother CPR three times in an attempt to save her life. But Hilary died in her daughter's arms. The little girl knew her mother trusted Pancho Kohner. She called him. Pancho went immediately to the apartment. Hilary was dead. Hilary's dog Bobo guarded the body, snarling and growling at anyone who came into the room. Katrina was hysterical.

Charlie and I raced in shock to Hilary's small apartment. The scene was tragic. Katrina, a blanket around her shoulders, sat on a couch holding her dog. She was a skinny little black-haired girl with huge brown eyes. She looked much younger than fourteen. She sat there whimpering.

Every now and then surges of strength surfaced. She made demands.

"I want my mommy's things. I want my dog. I want my cats. I want everything here in the apartment."

"Everything is yours, Katrina. You will have everything," I assured her.

This was awful. I walked into the bedroom. Hilary was lying on the bed. I looked at my friend for a long moment. I knew her last thoughts and fears had been for her daughter. I'll take care of her, Hilary, I promise you.

We hastily packed a small bag, took her dog, Bobo, and went home. We couldn't find the cats.

I had met Katrina only twice, but I felt I knew her. I certainly knew Hilary well, knew what she would have done. I tried to step into her shoes, to become Hilary for Katrina. For a year that was my top priority, to give Katrina the feeling she had a woman in her life who would care for her and love her.

The first few days were a nightmare. Funeral arrangements were made. I went to look at Hilary before Katrina did. Katrina insisted on seeing her mother one last time. It was to be an open-casket ritual. I looked at Hilary. Her face was made up in a way that did not seem quite right. I had brought her makeup with me and gave it to the mortician, telling him to make corrections. I redid her hair, pulling it forward over her brow the way she used to wear it. She was dressed in a pink-cotton dress her daughter had chosen. Katrina provided jewelry she knew her mother loved. She put snapshots of her mother and herself into the casket, saying, "I want Mommy to have them."

I held Katrina while she sobbed. "I want my mama. I want to be with Mama. Why did it have to happen? We were so happy."

Katrina had been her mother's life. Hilary loved her daughter with a passion. She put her first, before herself in all respects. Indeed, the message machine on her telephone said, "This is the answering service of Katrina and Hilary Holden." It demonstrated for Hilary that it was Katrina's home first and hers second.

The year went by. Katrina grew stronger. A basically happy girl, she did well in our family. Katrina and my daughter became close. Zuleika enjoyed having a sister near her own age in the house.

Having a new member of the family brings stresses of its own, but having a new teenager to raise and provide for was a bigger stress than anybody could anticipate. Charlie was wonderful. He opened his heart fully to Katrina. I was grateful. I wanted her, and it would have been hard on me if Charlie had been less than one hundred percent behind me. Blending a new personality into our home did pick up activities and responsibilities.

Paul, Tony, and Suzanne were living away from home now, so there was room for Katrina. When we received that tragic phone call, the first person we called was Paul. We asked him to come to the house and stay with Zuleika while we picked up Katrina. Zuleika and my youngest son, Valentine, sensed the disturbance and unease in the house. They awoke. The three of them—Paul, Valentine, and Zuleika—held a meeting. They decided to ask Charlie and me to take Katrina in and let her become part of the family.

I was glad my children accepted the newcomer with such open hearts and generosity. I did my best to fill Hilary's shoes. It was difficult for Katrina to adjust to becoming one of a large family, accustomed as she was to comprising her mother's entire family. In spite of this, though, she blossomed. From May to December, I watched the little waiflike girl bloom and grow into a lovely young woman.

Christmas of that year, 1982, came. My brother, John, and his family joined us in Vermont. I worried that Katrina's first Christmas without her mother might be difficult, but we got through it. I planted a tree for Hilary, a weeping willow because it was Hilary's favorite, and had a bronze plaque engraved:

Do not stand at my grave and weep;
I am not there. I do not sleep.
I am a thousand winds that blow.
I am the diamond glints on snow.
I am the sunlight on ripened grain.
I am the gentle autumn's rain.
When you awaken in the morning's hush,
I am the swift, uplifting rush of
    quiet birds in circled flight.
I am the soft stars that shine at night.
Do not stand at my grave and cry;
I am not there. I did not die.

Anon.

Mother's Day came and went. We decided to take flowers to her grave on Hilary's birthday. But it happened to fall on a national holiday and when we arrived the cemetery was closed. We broke into Hillside Memorial Cemetery. Katrina, Zuleika, and I, with Charlie's able assistance, climbed a six-and-a-half-foot wall. I stood on Charlie's shoulders, which was fine for scaling the top of the wall, but jumping to the ground on the other side was both perilous and hilarious.

I landed in a heap, saying, "Hilary, I hope you appreciate all the trouble we've taken to bring these flowers."

Charlie, Zuleika, and I took a walk, leaving Katrina alone to spend a few quiet minutes.

When Katrina became sixteen we had a party for her at a discotheque. She hardly resembled the little girl who had come to live with us two years earlier. She had filled out; her hair had been cut in a fashionable bob.

At age seventeen she joined Charlie and me and a group of friends at the very formal, very chic Grace Kelly Memorial Ball attended by the first family of Monaco in Beverly Hills.

I loaned my lovely adoptive daughter a magnificent crimson taffeta ball gown and my best ruby-and-emerald necklace and earrings. She was easily the most beautiful girl in the room.

Until recently, Katrina would sit lovingly on my lap to tell me her troubles. Now that she's nineteen we converse like mother and daughter and two dear friends.

So when I say I have three daughters, I include my own dearest Zuleika, my stepdaughter Suzanne, and my adoptive daughter, Katrina Holden, although she is not legally adopted.

Now an excellent student at UCLA, Katrina is so firmly integrated into the family she has assumed every possible daughter and sister prerogative imaginable. I often find her zooming in or out of the house in a blouse or skirt that looks suspiciously like Zuleika's, or a sweater I could swear belongs to me.

I often think, "Hilary, I hope you can see her. I know you'd be so proud."

32
Cancer

There was hair everywhere, thick hanks on the backs of chairs, bird's nests on the carpets, hair piled wet and sodden, matted in the drains, sticking to my body in the shower and bathtub. I had only to scratch my head or lightly touch my brow and it fell out.

Then, overnight, there was no more. The fallout stopped. It had all disappeared, carried away by the vacuum cleaner, the Los Angeles sewers, and plastic-wrapped in garbage cans.

I was bald.

My hair had been sacrificed for a greater cause—my life.

It was 1984 and I had cancer.

Three rough-and-ready friends were to be my companions for six months. Their names were Andriamycin, Cytoxin, and 5-F-U. They knew their job and for it they exacted a heavy price—my hair, my energy, my vision, my hearing, and finally my fertility.

I paid them and I paid them.

Then, having poisoned my cancer cells as much as

possible without killing me, they departed from my life as swiftly as they had become a part of it, leaving me to battle the ever-present cancer cells alone and unprotected. I was no longer paying them, but nothing is for nothing. Now I began paying tribute to other gods with other specie—my peace of mind, my wounded body and psyche, my newly formed image of myself as a cancer victim.

I made up my mind to attack everything on the home front. First things first. I would regain my equilibrium by nurturing myself and encouraging peace of mind. I would retire with my husband to Vermont, there to heal my wounds and maybe help my fragile confidence as well. In that first year fear was a constant companion, an unwelcome reminder that now I was different. I was an unwilling member of a club, a mastectomy victim and a cancer patient.

Cancer robbed me of my youth, the warm, golden remnants of it. But I told myself I still had my life, my senses of taste and sight. My hearing, I knew, I had to make the most of. My favorite music and children's voices were fading. Already Val's deep voice was in the low register that made it difficult for me to unscramble. What he said often sounded like a rumbling mumble.

The drugs, Cytoxin, 5-F-U, and Adriamycin had left me with a constant ringing in my ears, which also made sound unscrambling difficult. I developed joint pain and my left hip had become unreliable. Pain was a constant.

In spite of this, I fought depression, as in the glorious days of my taken-for-granted youth. There were days of moody rebellion and tearful melancholy. But I was learning, through holistic training, to enjoy what was there for me and to carefully nurture what was weakening. I found meditation and visualization spiritually strengthening.

At times I felt rather like an old car for which it is no longer profitable to get new parts. But I told myself that with care I could travel many more miles if I would learn to take the hills slowly and cool off at the top.

My family soon accustomed themselves to my illness. It was surprising how quickly we all learned to live with it. And still, life went on.

33
Dread

Terrified he would lose the one person he was sure of in his life, Kier plunged farther and farther into the world of escape. Would this woman who had replaced his real mother be taken from him too?

He could not bring himself to see her suffer, perhaps waste away before his eyes.

Kier, now twenty-one, saw Jason's mother only three times during her illness. His first sight of her with cancer was in Cedars-Sinai Medical Center shortly after her surgery. It shot him into an orbit of darkness and insecurity. Only the numbing escape of alcohol offered temporary sanctuary, a cessation of frenzy. Only this filled the cavernous empty spaces and made the time pass.

Kier saw Jason's mother grow more emaciated, losing her hair and her appearance. He saw the disfiguring mouth sores that prevented her from eating and the haunted look in her eyes. It was more than he could handle to see the quiet resignation. She no longer questioned him searchingly about how he felt and what he was doing. She had given him up to save herself.

34
R & R

"No more stress, Jill," my surgeon Dr. Mitchell Karlan said the last time I saw him. "Take it easy. You're going to make it. Have a restful vacation."

I was full of anticipation; we were going to Vermont. It was a long flight for me—five hours to Boston. And since my recent experiences with cancer and its treatment, I had developed a fear of being shut up anywhere.

I boarded the plane, strapped myself into my seat, and wondered whether I should take a Valium. Knowing Charlie would strongly disapprove, I desisted and opened a novel instead. The flight was uneventful and my confidence increased as I found that I did not suffer even a tiny attack of claustrophobia.

On landing, we walked through the long corridors of the Boston Airport to our destination, Air New England, as it was then called—or Scare New England as some of my children dubbed it. The plane was small, propeller-driven, with a seating capacity of twelve. It had no toilet and was prone to chronic vibrations and thumps of mysterious origins. It also offered extremes of heat and cold. But since it was to be no more than a forty-five-minute flight, once more I girded my loins, walked across a freezing-cold tarmac, up six rickety metal steps, then, crouching low, I squeezed through the small hatchway into the tiny craft.

Ecch. I don't like flying in planes that size. Never have. Never will. I find I always have to urinate halfway to our destination. The vibration increases the discomfort, that and often having no reading matter except the back of an air sickness bag or directions on what to do in an emergency. Neither do much to ease my distress.

But this was a bright, starry night and the plane was not too crowded. I strapped my shoulder bag in one seat, my heavy topcoat in another. Charles deposited himself on the opposite side of the airplane. He rocked back in his seat as if to push it back before seeing a small sign that read THESE SEATS DO NOT RECLINE

He gave me a moody stare.

"They don't recline, darling," I said unnecessarily.

The sound of the propellers as we taxied to the runway drowned his reply, if indeed he bothered to give me one.

I spent the forty-five minutes gazing out the window remembering times past when Charlie and I frequently chartered one of these planes to take the entire family to our Vermont farm for summer vacation. The family then consisted of six children. Four boys, two girls, two dogs and a cat, all of whom sat in the twelve-seater. The children ate peanut-butter-and-jelly sandwiches and chattered excitedly about who would go down first to the woodshed and warm up his mini-motorbike. And who was capable of doing the longest wheelie. Valentine always won hands down in the wheelie department, but that didn't prevent Paul, Tony, and Jason from competing ferociously for the title.

Charlie was very much the boys' noble leader in those days, dressed in brown-leather windbreaker, sturdy blue jeans, and lace-up motorcycle boots. The boys dressed in similar attire and tried their hardest to walk, talk, and be as much like Charlie as they could.

I would sit in the back of the plane, holding the leashes of two large German shepherds, Daisy and Sara; a basket beside me on a seat held my Siamese cat, Polar. Zuleika, the cuddly little girl whose fingers were always entwined in my hair, sat with me. She lovingly called me Mama.

Suzanne, Charlie's oldest daughter, was fifteen and really fell between the two groups. She did not belong to the boys' group and she was not of an age to enjoy the simple kindergarten games Zuleika and I often pursued. I frequently read aloud to Zuleika, even on a bumpy, jostling airplane. And so I read, wedged in with the hot little girl and two drooling, panting German shepherds, and listening to the guttural howls from Polar, who complained angrily about her accommodations.

Above the din of laughter and chatter, I could nearly always hear the sound of my middle son, Jason, he of the glossy black hair falling below his collar, almost to the middle of his shoulders sometimes, his dark-blue eyes with the fringe of black eyelashes. Even as a member of the mini-motorcycle gang, Jason had flair. A red bandana tied rakishly around his neck and under his leather jacket a Rolling Stones T-shirt.

In the two seats ahead of Jason and Val were Paul and Tony, their heads deep in motorcycle magazines.

As I sat in the plane this night with Charlie, those days were far away.

We were met at the airport by our caretaker Chuck. I snuggled down in the passenger-seat corner of the station wagon, staring out into the darkness, waiting for the first sight of Zuleika Farm. It was not an easy house to see at night since, much to the shock of the local residents, I had painted our home what the natives call purple and I call heather. The color of the house matches the heather that blooms on the hill behind the house in the fall. But the locals, accustomed to red brick, white clapboard, and pale yellow, or perhaps dark green, threw up their hands in disbelief when word got around that I had painted the house what everyone agreed was purple.

But that was many years ago. Later when I attempted to repaint the house a subdued gray, again all the Vermont hands rose in the air in shock and dismay. They said, "But we like it purple. It matches the bloom on the hill behind the house."

The farm was purchased the year of Zuleika's birth. A writer friend of ours had rented a house in Woodstock, Vermont, and had told us of its beauty. One weekend we flew from Los Angeles to see for ourselves. We fell in love with the area. Charlie had wanted a place in the country to give the children a taste of freedom unavailable to them in Los Angeles. He wanted them to love the woods, fields, and streams the way he did. Charlie felt at home there. Vermont reminded him of his native Pennsylvania. It spoke to me of parts of England I had known as a girl. After many weekends of searching we came upon the five hundred acres that would become Zuleika Farm.

On arriving this night, I opened the door, jumped down onto the driveway, and stood for a few moments inhaling the soft Vermont air, looking at the sky with its myriad stars and, as luck would have it, a beautiful full moon. Then, as was my habit, I walked down the drive, across the wide green lawn, to the post-and-rail-fenced pastures to talk to the horses. A favorite of mine, Turtle, raised his head from where he grazed and stared at me through the darkness.

"It's me, Turtle," I said. "I'm back. I made it back again. How are you doing, old boy?"

He came over. I reached across the fence and stroked his neck, trying to pull his head close enough so I could inhale the warm, woodsy smell of this horse.

Charlie, impatient, called. "Come on, Jill. You'll catch cold."

So I bid Turtle good-night. "See you tomorrow," I said.

And inhaling as much of the clean crisp air as I could, I ran back across the lawn, up the flagstone path, and in through the door of my house.

I was home.

Six months earlier I thought I would never see this dearly loved house again. I walked through the breezeway with its hooked rug and into the kitchen. It is a wonderful way to start the day, standing at the sink filling a kettle with clean, sweet-tasting water from a well deep under the house, while looking out at the green lawns stretching to the woods on a beautiful Vermont morning.

Happiness filled me this night. I left the kitchen, removing my coat as I went, dropping it on the bench in the hallway. Then I entered my favorite room, the sitting room. It is here that I spend so many hours in my large oatmeal armchair with its own footstool in a corner. It is flanked by windows on either side, providing me with a view to my left and right. I also have a view of the room, which I furnished with care and love. The cream rug with a green-and-blue border was hand-loomed specially for the room. It covers a wooden plank floor.

The window ledges hold many personal mementos; ornaments given me through the years by friends and family are cheerful reminders of the many Christmases and birthdays spent in this house. There are photographs of all my family on ledges, tabletops, and mantelpieces—happy childrens' faces smiling out of antique silver frames, a very handsome photograph of my father taken fifteen years earlier. He shares my love of horses and in this photograph he is standing beside a large bay stallion.

The room has many windows and two fireplaces. It had once been two rooms, a wall having been removed to make it a long bright area with a view from three sides of fields, horse pastures and silver birches.

The many scattered pillows have embroidered mottos:

YOUR DOG LOVES YOU WHEN NOBODY ELSE DOES, says a bright red pillow on my chair; CATS ARE PEOPLE TOO says another with a green-and-red border; TO THE WORLD'S GREATEST DAD says the petitpoint cushion on Charlie's chair. The room is redolent of herbs and spices that I keep in pots.

I stretched and inhaled the scent of home. I was so lucky. I had made it through my six months of chemotherapy. My children were all happy and healthy and now I was to spend two weeks in my favorite place in the world.

35
Heartbreak

1985

The last words of *Life Wish*, which I had written during my illness in 1984, were: "I was going to face 1985 square on."

Well, it was now January of the new year and I was home. I smiled smugly to myself as I removed my serviceable Vermont walking shoes and wriggled my toes on the soft nap of the handwoven carpet. I was secure.

The telephone rang.

I heard Charlie pick up the receiver in the kitchen.

"Who?" I heard him ask. "Who?"

I left the room. It didn't seem as if the call were for me. I walked up the stairs on my way to the bedroom. But as I ascended the staircase something in Charlie's voice made me think the call had something to do with the children. It was the way I heard him say, "He's got what?"

I quickened my step and hastened into the bedroom to pick up the telephone extension. As I pressed the receiver to my ear I heard an unfamiliar voice say very clearly, "We found morphine in his blood. The kid is on the needle."

36
Purgatory

1985

My heart stopped. I heard Charlie say, "My wife's on the phone, Dr. Levis. Will you please tell her what you just told me."

My legs grew weak and I sat on the edge of the bed praying that what I suddenly knew to be true would not be verified. It wouldn't be true. It couldn't be true.

"I'm sorry, Mrs. Bronson. I know this is going to be hard on you; I'm a parent myself. But your son Jason is suffering from hepatitis B. He's very ill. I suggest that, since it is highly contagious, you and your husband go to the nearest hospital and take an immunization course to protect yourselves. I know you've been having chemotherapy. You may be very susceptible.

"Unless he goes into the hospital right away, I'm afraid for his life. The boy is in very bad shape."

"But, but, how? How . . . would he get . . ."

Doctor Levis cut me off. "I'm sorry I have to tell you this but I'm afraid I have no choice. We found morphine and cocaine in his blood. The kid's on the needle. He's an addict."

At first the words made no sense, *The kid's on the needle.* Jason's on the needle. But the words *He's an addict* came through loud and clear. Well, there it was, the thing I'd been most scared of—out in the open.

I could no longer listen. Waves of pain surged through my body. I was shaking. I hung up the phone. Doubled over with grief, I walked out onto the landing and clung to the banister rail, sobbing. "Oh, my God. Jason. Oh, why? How could you let this happen! Why, Jason!"

The bottom fell out of my guts. Jason, a junkie, a heroin addict. I had suspected he was using cocaine and maybe drinking too much. Perhaps during my darkest hours I had worried that he was an alcoholic. I would remonstrate with him: "Jason, please don't drink. Please. I beg of you."

"Don't worry, Mom. Please, you have nothing to worry about. I'm happy; don't worry."

It was easier to believe him, so I put my blinkers on again, put it out of my mind. After all, Jason had always been unique, always with a totally different energy from the rest of the family. For years I'd covered up his willfulness, refusing to hear a word against him, instinctively shutting up anyone who seemed about to tell me anything. I was his champion, his protector. No lioness in her den ever protected her cubs with more devotion or ferocity.

I stumbled downstairs back into the sitting room and sank into my chair, pulling my knees up, hugging them. I cried and cried. I couldn't speak. I took the writing pad beside my chair and a Ziploc bag of pens from a magazine holder. I wrote: "Pain. Pain. Too Much Pain. How can I stand it? I can't. I won't. Jason is on the needle. Jason, a heroin addict."

I suddenly knew what it meant when people wrote that someone's heart breaks. I felt as if mine were shattered. It gave me more pain and fear than when I learned I had cancer. I could fight for my own life. Now I knew I was called upon to fight for my son's. But even with all the energy and force I could muster, I realized I would get nowhere in this battle unless Jason fought even harder.

37
Hell

1985

My son was ill, and my very life was threatened by the onslaught of so much stress. I love all my children, but somehow the love I received from the others did not ease the anguish.

Jason had a straight-through connection to my heart. When he hurt, I hurt. His happiness was of paramount importance to me. I was powerless to control my feelings. I had tried to let go. And indeed, during the one long summer when I underwent chemotherapy, I did let go. It was let go or die.

Jason sensed this and stayed away. I later learned that during the protracted summer of 1984 he had overdosed on heroin and would have died had his girlfriend, Moira, not found him blue-white and foaming at the mouth in their apartment. She telephoned an ambulance and rushed him to the hospital.

Typically, Jason never paid the bill. By the time the bills had caught up with us many months later, it was too late for me to try to cover up for him anymore. His problems were all out in the open. The order of the day was survival, both for me and Jason. It was like having cancer twice over, going through the horror all over again. Only this time it was worse. We were fighting for our lives. I was fighting for my own life and Jason's as well.

I was so open and vulnerable, unable to fend off anything. Anyone with one hand and no effort could reach out and touch me.

"How can it be," I asked myself, "that one son can make me so sorrowful? I have so much to be happy about. A beautiful home, two other good sons, loving daughters, a good husband."

But all those blessings shrank beside the pain I felt when I witnessed Jason's struggle and confusion. All my instincts were working to find a way to make him better, to shield him from more pain. I told myself it wasn't that I loved him more than the others; it was just that he needed me more.

I could only think about saving his life, then blocking all exits, covering them up before his problems got out into the world beyond our family. This was difficult; so many people were involved. Jason had contracted hepatitis B, the variety usually contracted from dirty hypodermic needles or infected blood. Everyone who had come into contact with Jason had to be given gamma globulin shots. The people next door who had shared a marijuana cigarette with him, his girlfriend and her younger brothers, his younger sisters and their friends. Charlie and I in Vermont. The whole business was an ordeal of fear and humiliation.

For ten days in Vermont, from the night of our arrival until Charlie and I departed, we lived in hell.

During this time Jason, still under the influence of drugs, strutted about as if it were nothing. Groups of people would meet in the doctor's office to receive their shots, as many as a dozen at a time, with Charlie angrily, resentfully, footing the bills.

Jason was unrepentant and went about carelessly exposing more people to the virus, sharing a coffee cup here, a cigarette there. I was advised to remain in Vermont, as there was nothing I could do. I received all this terrible news by telephone.

At first no one understood that it was a rare strain of hepatitis, a junkie's disease, usually spread by needle. Everyone sympathized with Jason and dutifully turned up for their shots, wondering where he could have contracted such a disease.

It was then that the doctor, frustrated in his efforts to control the epidemic Jason was spreading, finally had no recourse but to telephone me and Charlie with information that my beloved son was irresponsibly spreading the virus.

The doctor gave Jason time to do something to help himself, to enter the hospital, to stop exposing everyone to the disease. But Jason, as the doctor put it, behaved as if he were the central character in a highly entertaining movie, a real bigshot. He didn't take the disease or his condition seriously.

Drugged out of his mind most of the time, he was uncontrollable, exposing and reexposing his younger sisters over and over again; entering the kitchen, handling the dishes, silverware, and food, despite the doctor's admonitions to stop such activities.

Zuleika and Katrina were given shots every day because of the constant exposure. They became increasingly upset and angry, almost hating Jason.

Zuleika telephoned me. "Make him move out, Mom. The shots hurt; he doesn't care about us at all."

Katrina was more understanding of my grief. She listened sympathetically as I sobbed on the telephone, but she agreed with Zuleika. "Jason's under the influence of drugs all the time," she said.

Finally, Jason committed himself to a private hospital for drug abuse and the real nightmare started.

The next day the telephone calls began. He wanted out.

He called six and seven times a day, desperate, pathetic calls. He was hurting. He was terrified.

Jason was in pain and I couldn't bear it. Charlie told him he'd better stay in the hospital and obey the doctors as he wasn't going to allow Jason to return to the Bel Air house.

Jason was broke and ill. He had nowhere to go. Nowhere to turn. He was in the hospital voluntarily and could leave at any time. But there was nowhere left to go except to his drug-addict friends. And they wouldn't help him now that he had no money.

Because of the damage to his liver from hepatitis, the doctors said they were unable to give him medication to ease his heroin withdrawal. He became angry and frustrated. He begged the nurses for something to ease the pain.

"You've got to help me. I came here voluntarily. I put myself in your hands. I want to be here. I want to get straight, stay sober. I want to stay, but if you don't help me, I'm going to walk."

The nurses were not authorized to give pain pills.

Jason called Vermont, his voice desperate: "Mom, Mom, oh, Mom. I can't stand it. Mom, please let me go home. I'll kick it there; I know I will. I just want to go home to my room. Mom, please, talk to Charlie.

"I'm sick, Mom, I'm so sick," he whined.

I begged him. "Try, try, try to handle it, Jason. I know it's terrible; but if you get through this, you can be so proud of yourself. It's one of the hardest things anyone's had to do—to go through the pain of heroin withdrawal."

"It is, Mom. It is. I can't stand it. I can't handle it. Please help. Make them give me something. God, I hurt so much. I'm sick, Mom." He began to cry. "I can't talk anymore, Mom."

Then he would hang up, leaving me desolate.

Charlie tried to comfort me, but I was unreachable, imprisoned by grief.

"Jason," I would call. "Jason! Oh, how could you? How could you? My God. Oh, my God!"

I would lie beside Charlie in our king-size bed, my body curled up in a ball, my knees pressed hard against my chest.

Charlie tried to console me. "Jill," he would say gently. Then more firmly, "Stop it, Jill, you're going to hurt yourself."

But I could not stop. Charlie suffered mixed emotions. He was upset about Jason, but his overriding feeling was a terrible anger at the boy for letting this happen, for hurting me this way. He believed I had spoiled Jason. He said I had done nothing but lavish love and understanding on my son.

Charlie's rage was murderous. He said it was unfair, the shock of being a cancer victim, the amputation of my breast, all those months of chemotherapy, and now this.

"You don't deserve it, Jill," he said. "You've been told you're a bad statistic, that you shouldn't have stress. You don't deserve it."

Charlie could do nothing but witness my awful grief and rage inwardly at the cause. He could see how fragile I was becoming. My nerves were frayed, my hands shaking. I began to lose weight.

My husband would persuade me to leave the house for a drive in the beautiful Vermont countryside, but all I could do was stare out the window and weep. I mourned as if my son had died. I couldn't imagine living the rest of my life knowing that Jason could do it once more, go back to the needle, risk his life, knowing that one day I might get a phone call telling me it was all over, that Jason had died. I knew that ninety percent of drug addicts go back. I mourned.

We would return to the house after outings to find the telephone ringing and a desperate, abusive Jason on the line. "I'm leaving, Mom. I can't take it. I can't stand it here. It's nothing but a crock of shit. They're not giving me anything. They're all bastards. They're all fucking bastards."

Then once again I would summon all my strength, using

every part of my being, to buy time, to will him to stay in the hospital. I'd plead and cajole him into sticking it out, while all the time he cried like a baby.

"All I see is death, Mom. All around me. Just death and blackness. You don't understand; you don't know what it's like. I want to die. I won't make it."

"You've got to fight," I pleaded. "You're so young. The world is beautiful. There is so much you haven't done, so much to see. Please, Jason, I'm fighting so hard for my life; fight for yours, please, Jason."

I called the hospital doctors. "Can't you give him something?"

But they were afraid, saying, "He's got so much liver damage as it is; we can't give him painkillers."

I called Ray Weston who told me, "Whatever you do, Jill, don't kick this kid out. He'll die. He needs love and support to get through this."

Dr. Ron Gershwin at the hospital reiterated Ray's advice. "He needs love and support. Don't just dump him in some rehabilitation camp; he won't survive. His life is threatened."

Moira visited him and then called me. "He's threatening to leave the hospital," she said.

At eighteen and with dark hair and huge brown eyes, Moira began fighting for Jason in the only way she knew how. She used an old cowboy trick and took away his shoes to prevent him from leaving the hospital. Then she took his clothes. She hid his car and emptied the wardrobe in his room at home in the event he should go there.

Moira visited Jason every day and often called me in Vermont in frustration and anger. "Why doesn't he understand he needs help? Why does he talk about leaving?"

Then one day Ray Weston called from the hospital and asked both Charlie and me to get on the line.

"Thank God I came to the hospital today," he told us.

"When I arrived Jason was standing outside in pajama bottoms. He was barefoot with his friend Moira."

Jason had broken out and made it to Rangely Street in Hollywood, heroin row, where the junkies go to make a score. Sick with hepatitis and unable to stand the pain of withdrawal, Jason had one thought in mind when he escaped. A drug score, which he fixed up on the street. Then he called Moira to pick him up.

It was at that moment Ray arrived. Being well connected with the hospital, he managed to get Jason readmitted. Then Ray reviewed my son's chart and concluded Jason's case had been mishandled. Of course he should have been given medication to deal with the pain. But the medication would have to wait until Jason dried out from the fix he had just obtained.

Ray said again, "Don't give up on this kid. If you do, he'll die."

Not needing to hear this and unable to speak anymore, I hung up to watch Charlie's reactions to these words.

Jason continued his angry, manipulative, pathetic phone calls. "Hang on, Jason. Hang on for two more days. I'm coming home. I'll take care of you out there."

"I don't think I can, Mom. I can't hold on any longer."

I was terrified. "You must, Jason. You must fight. Please darling, I love you so much. I need you. I need my son. I want you back. Please hang on."

Then suddenly I gave up. With anger in my voice, I said, "If you go back to drugs, Jason, I will simply put up a gravestone, carve your name on it, and I'll pretend you're dead. Do you hear me, Jason? I'll have your name engraved on a tombstone. Good-bye."

Charlie got on the extension to berate the boy. "Do you hear what you're doing? Can you hear what you're doing to your mother? I'll tell you something, you little son-of-a-bitch, if this gives her cancer again, I'll get you. Do you hear me? I'll get you, Jason. She's my wife and you're hurting her. You better stick it out there and quit torturing my wife."

Then Charlie hung up.

Those calls took a toll on both of us. I cried every night, and Charlie became furious every night.

I begged Charlie, "Be good to him. He wants you, Charlie. He wants *you*. He needs a father."

"No, he doesn't. He's a selfish son-of-a-bitch, a selfish, self-indulgent son-of-a-bitch."

"Please don't talk that way. You don't understand him. I'll die if you hurt him and drive him to drugs again. Don't drive him away. Love him, Charlie, please."

Hysterically, I would pound my fists on the walls until my knuckles bled. I wanted to inflict pain on myself, anything to distract me from the dreadful pain I felt in my heart.

At times, when Jason felt stronger, usually after being given a sedative, he sounded more like himself. "Don't come home, Mom," he would say. "I don't want you to see me like this. Don't come home."

But a few hours later, strung out with pain and waiting for his next shot, he would be crazed, threatening to kill himself. Those declarations seemed to give him relief, but it was killing me. I couldn't sleep. I couldn't eat or control the dreadful shaking in my hands.

Ray was concerned for my health and advised me not to come home. "There's nothing you can do, Jill. This is something he has to do by himself. Stay where you are."

"I can't. I have to come, Ray."

Charlie agreed with the doctor, but I begged my husband, "Charlie, please, let's go home. I can't bear it."

I called the other children to say, "I love you. I'll be home in two days. I'm cutting my vacation short."

They had been so sweet when they kissed us good-bye. They knew it was a much needed two-week vacation.

"Have a good time. You've earned it."

They had been through the grueling ordeal of my mastectomy and illness. Now at last my hair had grown back from the chemotherapy-induced baldness. And I was released from the dreaded intravenous injections of nauseating anticancer drugs. Charlie and I were free to travel, to lick our wounds, to be together.

But it was not the second honeymoon we had hoped for, learning one of our children was a drug addict. It had a corrosive effect on our relationship. It was as if we had suffered a death in the family. We raged impotently and slept very little. Lack of sleep and the constant conflict made us both raw emotionally. Our eyes burned, our bodies ached. Unlike death there was no finality. We knew we would be living with this for a long time; at least until the other shoe dropped, and I prayed it never would.

We ate desultory dinners, often a frozen TV snack, and then after an evening of telephone haranguing, desperate pleas, and weeping, we would climb the stairs to our bedroom silently, lie down, neither one of us having the spirit or the emotional energy to speak of the family tragedy.

Jason was on my mind constantly. I imagined him writhing in torment, bathed in perspiration. His cries of "It hurts, Mom. It hurts" echoed constantly in my ears. I remembered the little boy. It was him I pictured suffering, not the man he had become. It was my baby that was hurting.

The emotional pain was depleting my healing resources and I knew I had to do something about it if I were to withstand this attack. I thought back to a time nine months previously when I was going through an assault of another kind. Then the enemy was within—cancer cells were the invaders. I had fought and was winning. But to help put everything in perspective and to stop feeling isolated I had daily written pages that became my book, *Life Wish*. It had helped me then. Maybe it would help me now.

Two or three mornings before I left Vermont, unable to

sleep and tired of staring at Charlie's slumbering back, I crept quietly out of bed.

Stealthily, so as not to wake my sleeping husband, I lifted the old iron latch on the bedroom door and crept down the stairs to the kitchen. I filled the copper kettle and stood, bare feet chilling on the blue-and-white tiled floor, waiting for the first burst of steam. I looked at the wall clock; it was five-thirty on a cold, gray morning. Turning, I saw my reflection in the window over the stainless-steel sink. God, I looked forlorn. There were dark shadows under my eyes, and my hair was in wiry disarray. The two furrows between my eyes gave me an expression of deeply etched pain.

Suddenly, the kettle gave a sputtering squeal. I grabbed it off the stove before the squeal became a shriek. I made my tea, taking it in trembling hands, trying to draw warmth from the mug as I walked into the cozy little sitting room.

I looked around with tired eyes at the attractive room. Smiling children's faces greeted me from out of hand-painted enamel frames that stood on the mantelpiece over the deep fireplace. My Siamese cat Polar greeted me from the deep confines of a beige chair. "Yup, yup," she said as she yawned. Even in the damp chill of the morning, it was a warm, happy room. A homemaker had put this room together with love and care. That was the statement it made, the one that I had in mind when I decorated it.

I pulled my blue-velvet robe more tightly around me, trying to keep out the chill. Another nearly sleepless night. I wondered how much longer I could go on this way, awaking at dawn, eyes swollen from crying, shoulders aching. I cracked my neck, trying to unclench the tight fist of tension. I felt isolated, numb with misery and fatigue.

"Oh, Jason. Oh, Jason."

My inner resources had been tapped to the limit. After cancer I thought I would never again be afraid of fear itself. But now, only six weeks after my last treatment, I had thought all I had to handle was every cancer victim's constant worry—a possible recurrence. No, for a different reason, I found myself in the same terrifyingly familiar situation. Here I was clawing my way to the surface of an oozing, emotional bog, the pain threatening to drag me under.

There in my exhausted brain was the thing I had been most afraid of. I could see it lying before me, dark, glistening like a lump of raw liver, a squirming mass of maggots at the bottom of a hole scratched by a mangy old cat. Repulsed, yet compelled, I looked long and hard.

"I'd need a fucking jackhammer to cover it up this time, cat," I said to Polar.

The situation demanded self-confrontation, complete honesty. I took a big gulp of the tea, rubbing my fists childlike against my eyes. Then I straightened my back, flexed my muscles like an old workhorse accustomed to heavy loads, and decided to start before I hastily scraped over the hole as I had done so many times before, unable to face the probing and dissecting that leaving it open would entail. My chest hurt from too much sobbing. I hadn't the strength or the heart to fight with myself any longer.

I sat down tiredly in my big armchair and turned to what I had relied upon for the last year of my life to keep my mind from splintering into a million spiky shards like a fine glass brandy snifter in the grip of a clumsy hand. I gave myself up to the ritual as, with a deep sigh, I reached into my pocket for my spectacles and prepared to write my way out of the mess.

Automatically, I opened the wrapping on a new stack of legal pads. First, I had to relieve the pressure, lance the festering abscess, let go, center myself. I started writing in bold slashes with a black felt-tip pen. This was the real work, the digging, searching, and just plain brain frying. Later I would dictate my notes to a tape player, editing, punctuating, and elaborating as I read. That was fun. But now it was difficult. I sat deep in thought, my surroundings fading as I slipped away into a world of my own.

My husband came into the room, recognizing the signs, the scattered paper all over the footstool, the plastic bag full of different-colored felt-tip pens.

"Good morning," he said. "Jesus, it's cold in here."

I looked up almost angrily over the top of my glasses. "What?"

He repeated levelly, "Good morning. It's cold in here."

"Oh, yes, good morning, Charlie." I watched him, feeling somehow almost guilty about the temperature of the room.

I hacked my nervous cough, clearing my throat unnecessarily before saying, "I'm starting a new book."

"I can see that." He looked concerned. "Do you think you're up to it? I mean, it won't take too much out of you?"

He hunched his shoulders. "Anyway," he continued. "What are you going to write about this time?"

"Jason and Daddy."

Charlie groaned and covered his face with his hands. "Oh, God."

Charlie is an extraordinarily private person who values the anonymity of his family life.

I became defensive. "Well, it's either that or go crazy. I've got to try to put my brain in some sort of livable order on the subject."

"Oh, God, please leave me out of it this time. You only write from your point of view. It's not fair to me."

"Well, I'll try, but Charlie, you do happen to be married to me, so it's almost impossible. Anyway, I've told you it's not going to be about you. It's about Jason and Daddy."

"Oh, shit," he said.

I slammed down my pen and pad. "Well, what the fuck do you want me to do? Charlie, what do you want me to be? A quiet, dignified woman or perhaps a dead wife? Why can't I be me, just a woman who writes?"

I took a cheap shot, why not, I thought, I've earned it.

"Charlie, perhaps I'll sidestep death from stress-induced cancer by writing about my problems."

That subject was an old one. Charlie's attitude was automatically fixed, his dialogue predictable. "Goddamn it, Jill, why does everything have to be you? I'm sick of pussyfooting around. All you think about is your feelings and to hell with everything and everybody else."

He looked at me murderously, his eyes slits. "Your feelings, your cancer. Do you have to have everything you want, and do I have to go along with it just because you've got cancer?"

I had heard it all before.

"I'm not going to play this morning, Charlie, so since it takes two to tango, you're up a gum tree. You better just go and get yourself some coffee and leave me alone."

He stared ominously. I backed off a step.

"I told you, I'm not writing about you. Oh, for crying out loud, Charlie, go away; I don't need this from you just now."

I felt myself beginning to fragment. "Charlie, please, not this morning. I'm too tired. We're both too tired."

This morning was getting off to a nasty start.

"Let me write. Let me breathe, please. Don't do this. Anyway, it's probably never going to be published. Please let me alone. Go and have your coffee. Be nice. Drop it, please."

Charlie left the room, made his coffee, and went back to the bedroom to drink it. He was not accustomed to having people question his authority. He'd fallen in love with me for my English reserve, youthful prettiness, and femininity. He couldn't handle it when I stood up to him this way. It wasn't what he'd married or what he wanted from a wife. He'd been accustomed to having his own way for a very long time now. I used to obey all his orders, cater to him, and go along with his moods. But since my illness I had changed, so his life was changed. I was not so malleable. I seemed to him to be developing a quarrelsome, selfish independence. His life was being disrupted.

I stared at the yellow-lined paper. Charlie had upset me, hurt me. I waited for the emotions to pass. I rubbed my eyes again with both fists, then studied the paper, gathering my concentration. As I did, pictures began to emerge as though from a crystal ball, sharp and clear as when they had happened. As the memories came flooding back to me, I picked up my pen and, narrowing my eyes almost automatically, I began to write.

A few days later Charlie, although he disapproved and wanted to keep me away from the whole scene, finally gave in to my pleas that we leave for Los Angeles to see what we could do to help Jason. With heavy hearts we shut the house and flew back to California. I was nervous and jittery the whole time. It was as if the plane could not fly fast enough for me.

38

Clean-up

1985

On arrival from Vermont, Charlie and I learned Jason had fled the hospital again. Technically, he should have been through most of the physical withdrawal, but he was still dangerously ill. He was bright yellow with hepatitis and very frail. Jason believed we would not allow him back in the house. He had broken out of the hospital and had gone to stay with an old friend.

The friend called. "He's terribly ill, Mrs. Bronson. I think Jason should be back in the hospital. He's in pain all the time, and he looks terrible. What should I do?"

"Bring him home," I said.

I prepared Jason's room with as much care as I had when he was a little boy recovering from mumps and measles. Fresh sheets, juice, and a jug of water on the bedside table. Everything neat and orderly.

I had anticipated the worst; all the same, I was shocked at Jason's appearance. In the ten days since I had seen him he had become emaciated. His eyeballs were yellowed from hepatitis; his skin was covered with sores; his hands shook even more violently than my own; his eyes were black-shadowed and burning with fever.

He was obviously terrified. And while he could look at me, he couldn't meet Charlie's eyes.

"Hi, Mom."

"Oh, hi, baby."

I stretched out my arms to hold him but Charlie restrained me.

"No, Jill. No contact. You can't afford to catch hepatitis. He's still highly contagious. Go to your room, Jason."

"I love you, baby," I said.

"I love you too, Mom," Jason replied.

He walked slowly, swaying as he went, his legs occasionally buckling.

"I feel so bad about this," Jason said.

He started to cry and I followed him into his room.

"Get into bed, darling. Oh, Jason, I can't believe it. I can't believe you're a junkie."

Through his tears, he said, "Mom, I wanted to tell you so many times. I was so ashamed. But you see when you're a junkie, you hate yourself so much that the last thing you want to admit is that you're a junkie, that you're addicted. But I wanted to tell you."

I searched my son's face. "Whatever made you do it? I don't understand. I've had so many drugs because of my illness I can't understand how someone can use drugs for recreation. How could you be so self-destructive?"

"Well, Mom, to tell you the truth, the first time I did it, I didn't know. I thought I was snorting cocaine, but they had cut it with heroin. And the next time I just did it for a lark."

I began to cry. "Jason, I feel so responsible. It must be my fault somehow."

Jason gave me a sharp look. He put his hands on my shoulders and gave me a shake. "Don't say that, Mom. Don't ever say that. It's not your fault. It's all my fault. I was stupid. Dumb. It has nothing to do with you. Nothing at all. Don't ever feel guilty."

We had our arms around each other. Now we were both crying.

"I'm so sorry, Mom. So sorry."

The horror notwithstanding, I felt better that Jason was home in his own room again where I could see him and do things for him. He was sober. It had been a long time since we had talked this way.

The next day Ray Weston arrived with a suggestion that Jason should see a psychiatrist who treated patients addicted to heroin and morphine.

"I think you should take Jason in tomorrow, Jill. You and Charlie should go with him."

Ray left some medication, saying, "You keep it and give it to him for the pains in his legs and the shaking. But only one every four hours."

Jason was shaking pitifully. He was so thin his clothes just hung on him. He hadn't eaten for days. Food wouldn't stay down. His stomach was sucked up and knotted with cramps.

The following day Charlie and I took him to Dr. Shapiro's office. The psychiatrist told me all the reasons why Jason had his problem. I thought I knew everything, but Dr. Shapiro laboriously described Jason's character in detail. He said he was cunning, spoiled, insecure, devious, and had a low self-image. He needed love and reassurance. He needed his family.

I wondered if I could sit through this. I put my head in my hands. I was weak. I didn't think I could handle it. It was frustrating to hear all the things I already knew, and I said so.

"Okay, Mom, okay," said Jason. "Dr. Shapiro's just trying to help me. Okay?"

Dr. Shapiro agreed to accept Jason as a patient with the proviso that he submit to a urine test once a week. Jason agreed.

"But can't you give me something for my head?" he asked the psychiatrist. "And my legs hurt terribly."

Jason sat there waggling and shaking his legs, shifting in his seat. He was sweating. His black hair stuck to his head in wet clumps.

Charlie said very little. He was morose. His shoulders were hunched. His hands were in his pockets. I wanted Charlie to show compassion for Jason, to tell him he loved him. But Charlie wasn't ready for that yet. He was still too angry.

We drove home in silence. That night Jason became more ill with ear and throat infections. Dr. Shapiro prescribed medication. At midnight I entered Jason's room to give him the medicine.

I found my son prowling restlessly, saying he couldn't stand the pain.

He needed something. He needed heroin.

I became exasperated. I was exhausted myself. "You've got to stand it. You can't have anything. I've given you everything the doctor said you could have. There's nothing else."

Jason was sullen. He glowered at me when I left, saying, "Try and get some rest."

I returned to his room later to find the door locked. I didn't like that. It hadn't been locked before. I pounded on the door.

"Just a minute, Mom; I'm putting on my clothes. Just a minute, okay?"

It took him a while, but Jason opened the door.

I was suspicious. "What have you been doing? What have you got? What have you stashed in this room?"

"Nothing, Mom. For God's sake, nothing. Leave me alone. You told me to rest. Well, I'm sleeping."

I had no choice but to trust him, so I returned to bed in desperate need of sleep.

"Good-night, Mom," Jason called. "See you in the morning."

The next day he was worse. He ate hardly anything. He sat in his room, shaking and chain-smoking cigarettes. He was in too much pain to visit Dr. Shapiro for therapy. It was a nightmare. Jason was repentant and anxious to stay sober, but the hepatitis was virulent. His craving for drugs grew worse.

I nursed him, babied him, and kept constant vigil at his bed, running down my own health, much to Charlie's fury.

Then one evening, despite my request that Jason not lock his door, I found his room bolted. After I had pounded for several minutes he opened up. It was obvious he had managed to get hold of some drugs. He must have a stash in his room, although Charlie and I had carefully stripped his bedroom, shaken it down before he came home.

I entered the room and stood for a moment; then with the unerring instinct of a police dog I walked straight to his curtains, reached down to the space between his wall and the bedside table, and picked up a large bag of marijuana.

"This is the last time you'll see this!" I said. "I'm going to flush it down the toilet."

"No! Mom! Don't do that. It's prime stuff. Five hundred dollars."

He was also naked and seemingly unaware of the fact. He sat on the edge of the bed, his speech slurred. I watched horrified as my naked son began laboriously to put on a pair of terrycloth socks, the kind I had bought for him since he was a toddler. He murmured incoherently to himself.

"What are you doing?" I asked.

He was surprised that I would ask such a question. "I'm putting on my socks. I don't want to catch a chill."

I couldn't answer. I could only stare. Jason had nearly killed himself and now he was worried about getting a chill.

Addicts are clever. I remember a doctor from the care unit telling me, "Addicts only live for the drug. They are devious, manipulative liars. Don't trust him. Watch him carefully. Remember he will die if he does further damage to his liver."

I looked on helplessly as Jason sank further into the world of hallucination.

Now, naked and smoking an invisible cigarette, he seemed to think he was in a restaurant. In fact, he was ordering dinner for both of us.

As if in a nightmare, I went along with it.

"What would you like?" he asked. "I'm having fish and Perrier water.

"No," he said to an invisible waiter, "we don't want wine."

Jason turned to me primly. "I don't drink; it's bad for my liver." He took another drag on his invisible cigarette and stubbed it out in the invisible ashtray beside him on the invisible table.

Now his mood changed. He looked at me with wide, calculating beautiful eyes. Then he began to whine in the drug addict's patois: "I'm sick. I'm hurting bad. Please, you've got to help me. I want you to go to Rangely Street, to Carl's market. Go to the back of the market and ask for Stan. There you can buy the stuff. Stan will cut it for you. Only I don't want you to go alone. Take him."

He gestured to an invisible man standing beside me. "Take him with you. Don't go alone."

Then in a stab of reality and an awareness of who he was talking to, Jason said, "Oh, Mom, I hurt so bad. I'm sorry. I didn't want anyone to know. I wanted to kick it on my own. I went for ten days, Mom. Then one day I was driving and my system started to reverse itself. I lost control of my bowels. The pain was so bad I had to get the medication."

Jason called heroin *medication*.

As he spoke there was a film of perspiration all over his body. His eyeballs were bright yellow and he was shaking with such force the bed was moving.

"Oh, Mom. Mommy," a whine now. "Mommy . . ."

I could stand it no longer. I gathered my son in my arms and rocked him as I had when he was a baby.

"Mommy loves you, Jason. I'll never let anything hurt you. I'll never let anything hurt you. I love you so much. You know that."

Jason stepped back into delirium.

I went upstairs to my husband.

"He's dreadfully sick, Charlie. He should be in the hospital. We've got to put him in. We must do something. Call Ray Weston, please. Don't let him die, I beg you. Don't let him hurt. I can't bear it. Please, Charlie."

I screamed at him, "Do something!"

Then I ran back to Jason, who was now picking things out of the air, saying huge ants were crawling on the walls. He was calm and quiet but totally disoriented, in another world. A world where ants crawled the walls of his room and large flying things were in the air to be grabbed at.

At one point he walked into the wall, then turned around and urinated on the floor. I could only watch.

Ray Weston arrived, horrified.

"He's got to be hospitalized, honey. You can't keep him at home like this."

"I know, Ray. I want him to go."

Jason heard me and flew at Charlie, who stood in the doorway. "Please don't put me away. Please, please, please, Charlie. Dad . . ."

It was a cry from the heart.

Jason jumped on Charlie like a three-year-old, wrapping his skinny arms and legs around him.

Charlie held him tightly, tears in his eyes.

"It's not forever, Jason. I'll be with you. Come on now, let's get you dressed."

"No!" Jason screamed. "Don't shut me up. I won't go. I won't. Please don't lock me up."

I was in purgatory. "Jason, Jason, you must go; you're ill."

Charlie's eyes were agonized. "I can't force him, Jill, and I can't carry him. I won't let them come and put restraints on him. Let's wait until morning."

Ray left. We were in over our heads. Charlie went to bed and I spent a long sleepless night on the couch in Jason's room. He paced the floor and grew more incoherent. At one point I fell asleep from exhaustion. While I slept, he somehow cut his foot and walked through the house leaving a trail of bloody footprints behind. I awoke and followed the bloodstains in panic. They led to the front door. He was in the driveway, naked, searching the bushes that grew at the edge of the garden. He had cut his toe severely.

I brought him back inside, dressed him in clean pajamas and, heedless of all the warnings about handling his blood, I bathed and dressed his toe. Then I sat down and waited for daylight.

Jason was now far from the realm of reality. I knew he would go to the hospital meekly. He wouldn't know where he was going. There would be no more screams of protest, at least no audible ones. Only those in the cage of my mind.

The next morning, accompanied by my friend Alan Marshall and Charlie, we left the house. I clung to Alan's arm as Charlie half-carried Jason down the stairs. Charlie told me I wouldn't be needed and should stay at home. Jason did not know anyone was there anyway. Charlie and Alan climbed into my Ford Bronco and left for the hospital.

Jason, deeply incoherent, had no idea of his whereabouts when they led him off to an isolation unit. Jason had known Alan since he was three years old. But today he didn't know Alan was present. Jason had eyes only for Charlie. He clung to him, speaking only to Charlie.

Alan accompanied Charlie and Jason to the hospital room, wondering how much more we could take. However, no tragedy is without its humorous moments.

Jason suddenly looked over at Alan, who was sitting quietly in a corner, then swiveled his head to Charlie. Then back again to Alan. Then with an ingenious smile and a wink, Jason turned to Charlie and said, "Jesus, Charlie, for a minute I thought *that* was alive"—referring to a much-chagrined Alan.

Our exasperated friend said, "I don't think there's anything more I can do here." He went home, not amused by Jason's evaluation.

Jason remained in the hospital two weeks, during which time he was detoxed completely and recovered from hepatitis.

During his brief stay at home and despite my vigil, Jason had managed to ingest a large quantity of marijuana. The medical staff could only assume he had hidden the pot in his room somewhere and had eaten it while he was disoriented —eaten it as a child would eat a cookie. I later learned he had buried his stash beneath some bushes in a neighbor's garden.

I visited Jason every day, sometime accompanied by Charlie and once with Katrina and Paul. Tony visited often, and once he said, "I feel responsible somehow. I really took advantage of Jason when we were growing up because I was bigger and older."

I was amazed to hear this coming from my stepson. It was probably the most honest thing I had ever heard him utter about his relationship with his stepbrother. However, I also knew Tony was not responsible for Jason's addiction, and I told him as much.

After Jason's return home he began seeing Dr. Shapiro once a week. The doctor insisted that as part of his treatment Jason leave home, find an apartment and a job. In other words, find himself. Grow up. Charlie heartily concurred and I was forced to cut the apron strings and gnaw through the umbilical cord.

I tried to let go, but somehow it didn't seem realistic. How could he find a job and an apartment with no money and no real skills? I felt the pressure would prove too much for Jason. But I bowed to the professional's advice and life returned to normal on Udine Way.

Once away from home, Jason seemed to blossom. He found an apartment, moved in with his girlfriend, and found a job working for a recording studio, running errands, sweeping the floors after late-night sessions, and learning to work the mixing boards.

Still, I felt insecure about my son. I worried, but I had to admit Jason did seem to be doing all right on his own. I was lonely and Charlie was too angry and hostile to be much comfort. He was prone to bark at me.

The whole thing had taken a toll. We needed space and time to lick our wounds. Charlie and I grew apart, each retreating into a private world. Days would pass without any intimate or meaningful conversation.

Alan was a strong and helpful ally, even though I noticed a weakening and deterioration in Alan's own health. A warning bell rang in my head. I prayed Alan hadn't contracted the dreaded AIDS virus.

"Honey," Alan said one day, "everyone's got to do his own shit. Don't worry about me; I've got lots of energy. Nothing's going to happen to me. And leave Jason alone. Let him live his own life. Let him stand on his own two feet."

"But I miss him, Alan. I need him."

"You've got the others, and Charlie."

"I know, but somehow I feel so incomplete without Jason. I understand him. I'm linked to him somehow."

Alan looked at me. "Jill, it's killing him. Haven't you noticed? He has to get away from you. Let him be."

I stared at my friend. I wanted to say, "Shut up, Alan, what the fuck would you know about being a mother, or father for that matter? He's my son. I love him. He needs me."

The weeks passed. My book, *Life Wish*, was accepted for publication. Charlie and I relaxed and our homelife returned to normal. I began riding my horses, taking Zuleika to horse shows, listening to Katrina's stories about her boyfriends, helping the girls with their homework.

I didn't see much of Alan during this period. He developed a series of colds and remained at his home with his friend Jimmy. Then one day while I was revising my book, sitting in my favorite chair, Jason walked in. He looked well. He had gained weight. His skin was healthy and his eyes were clear. I gazed at him, feeling my heart soften around the edges.

My son had returned to me.

"How are you, darling?"

"I'm great, Mom. I just got myself a really neat job as a personal assistant for Richard Antony. I'm really happy. I start next Monday. How are you, Mom?"

I removed my glasses and rubbed my eyes.

"Come here, darling, let's be together for a moment."

Jason sat beside me. He looked at peace with himself. I feasted my eyes.

"You know, Mom, I've been thinking about you. You're such a strong, free spirit, but you're going through the same thing I'm going through. You're fighting for your own identity."

"Oh, wise one, you're right. How did you know? I need to be myself again, not an appendage to someone else. I need my own place. I'm nearly fifty years old, Jason. If I don't make myself happy now, when will I?"

"Don't think about your age, Mom. With you it means nothing; you're so beautiful."

"I don't, darling; but, God, I could have died last year. It would have been all over."

"How's the book coming?" Jason asked, inspecting the manuscript.

"Okay. I've broken the back of the rewrites."

He took one of my cassettes scattered on the floor around my chair and pushed it into my tape player. Immediately, Neil Young's "The Needle and the Damage Done" started. We listened to the song together.

Jason asked, "Do you mind if I have a cigarette?"

I smiled. "No, you can't give everything up at once. I know that."

I watched him smoke. We sat companionably listening to the music.

I caught you knockin' at my cellar door
I love you baby can I have some more
Oh, the damage done.
I hit the city and I lost my band
I watched the needle take another man
Gone, gone the damage done.

I sing this song because I love the man.
I know that some of you won't understand
Milk, but to keep from runnin' out.
I've seen the needle and the damage done
A little part of it, in ev'ry man
And ev'ry junkie's is like the settin' sun.

The song reminded me of Jason. That was the reason I had put it on the tape. Now, when it was over, Jason said, "Not anymore, Mom. Not anymore."

He finished his smoke and looked at his watch. "Got to

go, Mom. I really just came by to touch base and tell you I love you."

I watched my son walk out of the room, aware of his strength, recognizing that it had come through pain just as mine had. I had him back, and it felt good.

39

Tea at the Dorchester

1985

In the spring of 1985 Charlie was on location in England shooting a new film. Zuleika, Katrina, and I had accompanied him.

It had been twelve months since my surgery. I was confident and happy, although it was not yet possible for me to be totally without fear. It was taking time and patience learning to live with cancer. It's a primitive environment, the fight for survival. I had my ups and downs.

One day I discovered a lumpy condition in my left breast. I had examined myself so many times I knew every gland, vein, and small swelling. This day my entire breast seemed to be made up of lumps.

To distract my anxiety, I opened the large French doors of our suite at the Dorchester and stepped onto the terrace to be greeted by a charming view of a quaint narrow street. I looked down on gray slate roofs, red brick, and whitewashed chimney stacks. Over a wall I spied someone's back garden, washing on the line, with flowers and a green lawn. The evening sun shone on my face. The world looked lovely. I was overtaken by a compelling desire to give up worrying.

Just stop it, the incessant kneading and self-examination, the meditating and homeopathic pill-taking. Oh, to run out into that sunny London street and forget everything. But I wasn't ready for it. Not yet. To allay my fear of another malignancy, I made an appointment to see a specialist in two days. The lumps in my breast were persistent. There was a real possibility one of them was a group of cancerous cells clustering to rapidly grow into a tumor. If this were the case, time was of the essence.

Instinctively, I cupped my left breast in my hand. Poor breast, sitting bravely there on my chest without its mate, like an old maid on a park bench. If you can hang on long enough, I told it, I'll give you a new companion—a perfect man-made mate, impervious to time. As a matter of fact, my dear, I will give you a small lift to match your new partner. All will be wonderful. You and I, my dear breast, have a lot to stay well for.

It would be almost another year before I could get through several days without thinking about getting cancer. But now on that sunny terrace, the fear was very much in evidence, quite suddenly producing fearful swoopings and flutterings in my stomach.

I could not allow this to go on. My thoughts had turned spitefully around and attacked me. Was this an inner knowledge, the feeling of impending doom that I had experienced before my surgery?

My brain was a merry-go-round. I was close to losing it. I needed to unload on someone. The door to the suite opened. Charlie was home from work. He looked and felt awful. He had a dreadful cold. I couldn't unload on him. He had enough to handle.

I filled the big tub and Charlie took a bath. I cut up a melon and spoon fed him while he lay in my bubble bath. He had not eaten all day. He seemed feverish. He was ill and I was glad he accepted the melon after first expressing embarrassment over being spoon fed.

I did not share my personal concern with him. In the next two days my medical examination came and went. The English doctor said the lumps were mastitis or cysts, not at all uncommon. For now all was well.

I was well and ready for the tea party the girls and I had planned.

Bing-bong. The doorbell. Our guests had arrived.

My aunt entered first, limping badly from her left hip.

"Oh, Auntie, how good to see you. How are you?"

"I'm getting old, Jill. Getting old."

The words came out as dry as autumn leaves. Once a tall and striking woman, Auntie at eighty was frail. She was, however, still stylishly dressed in pale-green cashmere sweater, green-and-gray tartan pleated skirt, and a good-looking pin on her smart felt hat.

Saying her voice had rusted away with the years, Auntie spoke either in a whisper or she mimed the words, a sound escaping every other word or so.

My mother bustled sturdily in behind her, totally unlike my aunt in her demeanor. While Auntie seemed only a ghost of her former self, my seventy-eight-year-old mother still flashed with personality. Her hearty laugh, bright shiny eyes, inquiring expression, and challenging stance told the world this was still a woman to be reckoned with.

"Hello, Jilly," she said, as we met in the long corridor to the suite.

"Lo lo lo," a gruff masculine voice said. "Lo lo lo."

There he was. My father, white hair and mustache, ruddy, glowing face, eyes snapping with the excitement of seeing me. A short stocky figure sporting a brown tweed jacket and leather running shoes. In his left hand he firmly gripped a stout wooden walking stick. His right arm rested limply at his side, his hand tucked into his jacket pocket. He could not speak words, but by God, he made his presence felt.

He looked at me, his eyes boring holes into my face. I heard the unspoken question.

I gave the answer.

"I'm well, Daddy. I'm all right. It's all over."

"Ha ha ha." He laughed triumphantly. He could see I was fine. Ireland strength had prevailed.

I was not only recovered, but looking good. He carefully propped his stick against the wall. Then with his good arm he reached out to me. He touched my hair very, very gently with an inquiring expression in his expressive brown eyes.

"Yes, Daddy, it's all mine. It grew back thicker than ever."

I knew he was thinking of the chemotherapy and how I had lost my hair. He gave another triumphant laugh, his head thrown back this time. The laugh was aimed at the gods. Thought they could get an Ireland down, did they? Well, they had another think coming. His eyes sparkled.

"Ha, ha," he said, shaking his head with a gesture expressing disbelief tinged with pride. His eyes sparkled with tears.

"He's been geared up for this visit ever since he heard you were coming to England," said my mother.

"Yush," said my father. "Yush."

He still hadn't taken his eyes from me.

I helped him get seated in one of the comfortable green-velvet arm chairs. Zuleika and Katrina told my mother and aunt about all the things they had been doing in London. The excitement in the room mounted.

My father beamed, the patriarch, looking around at the womenfolk; his daughter, granddaughters, sister-in-law, and wife.

"Lo lo lo," he said, pointing to his jacket.

"Very smart, Daddy."

"John bought it for him last summer," my mother said in reference to my brother John.

"Lo lo lo."

This time the left hand flipped his necktie in the air.

"Oh, yes, Daddy. I remember. It's an old one of Charlie's. You look so smart. You're still a handsome devil."

"Yush," said Daddy.

My mother fidgeted.

"I had to trim his mustache before we left," she said. "I think I took too much off the sides."

"No, you didn't. He looks lovely. Most distinguished," I said. "But how are *you*, Mummy?"

My poor mother was clearly harassed, quite exhausted from handling my father and his excitement. The long drive to London from Sussex had been draining. There were pale-blue shadows on the transparent skin beneath her eyes.

My mother looked sharply at my father.

"Jack, where's your hearing aid?" she asked.

"Lo lo lo?" My father put his hand to his ear.

My mother raised her voice shrilly. "Your hearing aid! Oh," she added in exasperation, "you forgot to put it on. Now you won't hear properly and I will have to keep telling you what everyone is saying."

"Oh, Mummy, don't worry. It'll be all right. Let's order a light lunch."

But she wasn't finished. "Jack, where are your glasses?"

"Lo lo?"

This time the triumph faded from his eyes. He had forgotten them too. He had failed: hearing aid and glasses.

"Oh, well, not to worry," I said, buzzing for room service.

At this moment Daddy, with an up-and-down pendulum motion of his left leg, levered himself to his feet and disappeared into the bathroom.

My mother relaxed a little when he was out of the room. We sat together on the sofa. I hadn't seen her since the previous summer on the beach while I was undergoing chemotherapy.

"How are your feet, Mummy? Prisoners again?"

I was referring to the previous summer when it had been difficult for me to persuade my mother to take off her shoes and walk barefoot in the sand while she was visiting me in Malibu. She refused to bare those arthritic extremities, trundling along in socks, the toes of which became filled with sodden sand. Finally she had abandoned the sand-laden socks and I convinced her to bathe her feet in the California sunshine and the healing brine of the gentle Pacific, her embarrassment at her arthritically deformed feet finally forgotten.

"So far they haven't given me any problems. Touch wood. You do look well, Jill."

The waiter arrived and there was much excitement as everyone ordered lunch.

"Where's Grandpa?" Zuleika asked. "He's been gone a long time."

I went to see if Daddy was all right.

"Lo lo lo," said the voice from the bathroom.

He sounded in distress. I called to my mother, "I think he wants you."

My mother sounded so tired. She arose with effort and left the room. A few moments later she reappeared, signaling we had to confer.

"Jill, he's had an accident. His colostomy bag leaked on his underwear. Can you find him a robe? I'll have to help him change."

My God, this once strong, proud man hiding in a hotel bathroom.

"Oh, dear, what a shame," I said.

I found a short terrycloth hotel robe. We put it on Daddy, then pinned a towel around his waist for modesty's sake. Daddy was abashed.

"Don't worry, Dad, accidents happen. Come on out."

I asked our secretary, Sue Overholt, to buy new underwear. Daddy returned to the green chair. It was hard to keep his dignity, but he tried. He seemed to withdraw into himself, imagining he was not even in the room.

Zulieka and Katrina began a game of gin rummy with him to cheer him up.

Lunch arrived and a table was set up in the middle of the room. Daddy appeared to forget his troubles and everyone benefited from the nourishment.

Sue returned with a pair of flowered red, white, and blue boxer shorts. They were size large, but by no means the kind of large my father would find comfortable.

"What shall we do?" we whispered conspiratorially at the door. My mother heard us.

"We can't let him sit in the towel all afternoon. Let's wash his drawers," I suggested. "We'll dry them on the hot-towel rails."

Soon we had a clean pair of drawers. I rolled them in a towel to take out most of the water, then we began the drying operation. Sue sat on the floor with her hair blower while I held out the large white flannel underpants, which flapped in the breeze like a sail.

"Well, now I've seen everything," said Mummy, watching from her perch on the bed.

They dried in minutes.

I stood up. "Okay, let's get him dressed."

I had folded his slacks over the heated towel rail so they were neatly pressed and ready. Soon Daddy was once again his dapper self.

That was a close one, I told myself. What with no glasses, no hearing aid, and no underdrawers it would have been hard for Jack Ireland to greet his son-in-law with any semblance of personal dignity. But now fed and reclothed he was once again himself. It was just one of the many times during my visit to England that I marveled at my mother's fortitude and resilience and at my father's ability to maintain his dignity under the humiliation of his handicap.

During the next few weeks while Charlie toiled away on his movie, the girls, my parents, and I spent the time happily together. All too soon it ran out, and sadly we said good-bye to Grandpa and Grandma and Auntie Edie.

40

Vermont

After leaving my parents in England, we spent the rest of the summer in Vermont.

On my first day in the country I strolled down the winding road on our property to the big indoor riding arena. I stopped at the smaller of our two ponds and checked on Hilary's tree, the weeping willow. It was flourishing.

As I stood there, I found myself thinking how my auntie had aged. I thought she would not live very long and, indeed, she did not last out the year. Compared to my parents, she seemed devoid of that essential life force.

My grandmother, Sarah Eborn, gave birth to three daughters. It was my mother, her youngest, who was at her side holding her hand when she died. It was to my mother that she turned her head and asked quite clearly, "I wonder, where do Dollys go when they die?"

And although my mother was called Dolly, she took the reference to mean women as dollies. My grandmother wanted to know where women went when they died. It seemed she wasn't particularly interested in the fate of men.

Perhaps after a lifetime of caring for her own father, husband, and sons, heaven to her was a place where one no longer needed to cater to the needs, whims, and tyranny of the masculine sex.

Sarah's daughter Edith was seventy-five when she took photographs of Paul, Tony, Jason, Suzanne, and Valentine learning to skate on the pond a long time ago; but it was Jason who made her laugh. He couldn't skate. Instead of sliding on the blades like the others, he hunched his body and ran across the ice on the points of his skates, his heavy topcoat flapping. Auntie thought he looked like a little old man tippy-toeing over the pond.

Auntie was game that winter. She sledded down a hill on her belly like an eight-year-old. I like to remember her that way.

All that was left to me now were the memories and a bottle of Old English lavender water I had asked her to buy for me. I remember her saying, "Why do you want that, Jill? Whatever will you do with it?"

I replied, "I'll keep it here in Vermont, Auntie. It will always remind me of you."

I placed her gift where it still sits in the powder room. I never enter that room without picking up the dark green, oval-shaped bottle to hold under my nose to inhale once more the fragrance of my Auntie Edie.

My thoughts returned to the present. I walked briskly on to the barn that I consider my personal stable, as opposed to the big barn where I keep boarders and horses for sale. It's a six-horse barn, cozy and snug. I slid the large door open and entered. There were no occupants. I stood quietly, speaking aloud the names of each horse that had once inhabited the stalls: my favorite horse, Pat Hand, now gone, Limo, Rolls, Dennis, my very first horse. I inhaled the scent of sawdust, the aroma of the barn. I entered the tack room and gazed at the photographs, feeling the loss of power and ability, looking long and hard at Charlie's photograph. He was so strong and handsome under a thick layer of dust, sitting straight in his tuxedo on a galloping horse, a shot from the movie *Noon Until Three*. Again, riding hell-for-leather in only a loincloth, galloping recklessly on a gray stallion with a herd of wild horses in a shot from *Chatto's Land*. It seemed only yesterday.

It was an exhilarating summer, free of chemotherapy—a summer of lying naked down by the pond with Linda Harwood, fondly called "Pesty," who worked for Zulieka Farm West as a horse trainer, Katrina, thirteen-year-old Zuleika, her cousin Lindsay Ireland, and her friends Rachel and Marin. Lying by the pond, the young girls became accustomed to the sight of my Amazon-like scar. They were halcyon days, free from worry. A healing summer of sunshine.

My friend Susie Dotan spent two weeks with me, as did my sister-in-law Sandra and my brother John.

The days lazed by. And with good company, plenty of good books to read, my dogs and horses, my confidence in my health grew. I became less concerned with every ache and pain. And although the cancer monster still sat on my shoulder, I carried my burden more easily. The weight I could not and would never carry easily was the knot in my soul, the knowledge that my middle son was now and forever a drug addict. But for now, Jason was clean and I was taking a necessary respite from apprehension.

41
Jill's Birthday

1986

I was lying in my four-poster bed in the dressing room of the Bel Air house. My temperature at the last reading was 104 degrees as my immune system battled pleurisy and double pneumonia. In the midst of this swampy miasma, the telephone rang beside my bed.

"Hello, Jill," said the bright, upbeat voice of Pancho Kohner, the film producer. "Would you like to be involved as coproducer of *My Affair with the President's Wife*? We begin preproduction the second week in May."

Even in my stupor I could remember it was April, just one week before my birthday. Two weeks previously I had had a lumpectomy, which had probably brought on the pneumonia. I doubted I would be healthy in time for the film, but I punted and told Pancho to send me the script.

I liked the screenplay. All the same, I had doubts about working because deep chest congestion caused me to cough up blood clots. If it had been a movie I was watching and not my life, I'd have thought the heroine was not long for this world, a role that should go to a minor character. A star would not accept the part.

The night of my fiftieth birthday arrived and my temperature was still hovering at 102. Ray Weston took my pulse, frowned, and looked at a concerned Charlie, saying, "I've never known Jill so ill."

I stared at the chiffon party dress hanging from the rail of my four-poster, placed there for inspiration. I was determined to go to my birthday party.

Here I was at home with a huge party in my honor already in progress on the other side of town. It was being held at the Los Angeles Equestrian Center. Five hundred guests would be seated at their name-placed tables. Lighted trees and fairylike balloons, pink tablecloths and a huge birthday cake with a sculpted me in icing jumping my favorite horse Limo, were awaiting my arrival.

Almost everyone I had been close friends with, done business with or worked with, admired or fought with, had been invited. It wasn't every year one turned fifty, and a short time earlier it had been doubtful if I would ever celebrate my forty-ninth birthday.

I sat, hair awry, slugging cough syrup from an evil-looking dark-brown bottle with the aplomb of W. C. Fields, while all those around me were placating, trying to discourage me from thinking about the party. But I was determined.

One by one my houseguests came into my dressing room to show me their finery and to give me birthday gifts.

"We'll just go for a little while," they said, or "I'll just put in an appearance."

"Harumph, quite," I'd mutter as they kissed my fevered brow.

The last guest departed, as did the last child, my daughter dressed in borrowed finery, a black chain-mail Gianni Versace original. I watched my dress depart for the party, smiling to myself. At least four other of my gowns would be dancing on the floor of the Equestrian Center on the backs of my girlfriend Maggie, her daughter Debbie, Katrina, and my sister-in-law Sandra.

Charlie came in dressed immaculately. I sat up in bed hugging my knees and looked at him wistfully.

"Is there a limousine outside?" I asked.

"There is, baby, but I think you should stay here where it's warm."

"You go ahead, Charlie. You should be there. After all, they are our guests. Leave the limo here in case I feel better. Please?"

Charlie knew better. He knew me and saw the stubborn look in my eyes.

He said, "I'll wait for you."

I felt a silly childish grin spread over my face. "I feel ever so much better, Charlie," I said. "I'll go for only half an hour."

"I'll wait for you down in the study," he said, shaking his head in resignation.

Beads of perspiration formed on my brow as I secretly checked my fever therometer. My temperature was 102. Not so bad. It had been 104 all week. I bedecked my aching, insecure body in the pink-and-lavender chiffon beaded gown, ordered specifically for this party in healthier days, then threw an ankle-length white ermine coat over the top.

I looked at myself in the full-length mirror of my dressing room. A pampered, spoiled, fifty-year-old darling looked back at me out of carefully shadowed, butterfly-wing eyelids—what a package to thrash around in.

I studied the frothy apparition before me. She looked about as deep as a saucer. But how dare I make such an assumption about a woman who was on her feet, bloody but unbowed, after such a difficult three weeks? Nay, let's go back farther, a difficult twenty years. This was no fragile chiffon layer cake I was seeing; this was a heavier concoction, so give her a break.

A wracking cough sent me into a head-spinning, blood-spitting spasm of pain. Yuck. How typical—I would end my first half century dressed to the hilt, lying, as my husband had put it two nights previously, in the lap of luxury, ready to collapse.

My weak state infuriated me. Fuck this for a life; I needed some fun. So, sick as a dog, I went to the party, took off my shoes, and danced until one o'clock in the morning.

At the party Menahem Golan and Yorum Globus of Cannon Films saw me dancing like a dervish dressed in my beautiful gown, my eyes bright with fever. They thought I looked the picture of health. Menahem approached with a quaint suggestion.

"Jill, we would like to get into marriage with you."

I guessed what he meant, but I played coy. "I'm already married."

"No, Jill, we want you to play the first lady in the picture."

"Oh, my gosh." And here I was using up at least two weeks' energy in one night. I hid the brown bottle of cough medicine behind my back and accepted a fancily wrapped gift Menahem handed me.

"You don't have to do that," I said. "Are you sure you want me? I mean, I've been thinking of lots of actresses who would be wonderful in the role. Jaclyn Smith, for instance."

They were astonished. Nonplussed. Actresses rarely suggest another performer for a role they've just been offered. But it made Menahem and Yorum press harder. "But we want you," Yorum said.

Charlie joined our group. "What's going on?"

"We want her to star in the movie, if it's okay with you," said Yorum.

"Sure," Charlie replied.

"And so you don't think we are cheapskates, we have also given her a real present," Menahem said, indicating the package in my hand.

"Well, it's all settled," Yorum said.

My agent, David Shapiro, was spotted across the room by Menahem, who shouted, "Hey, agent! I want to make a deal."

"Well, baby," Charlie said, "it looks like you've got yourself a job. Do you think you're up to it?" He put his arm protectively around my shoulders. "Don't get cold; you're already sweaty. Go sit down and put your coat over your shoulders."

"I'm fine, Charlie, really."

I returned to the floor and danced with Jason and other male members of my family. I recalled *Life Wish* was due out in January of 1987 and this movie was scheduled to be released at the same time. It was fate. I could bring hope to many people with life-threatening diseases by being seen up there on the screen.

As I cut my cake and blew out the candles, I vowed to do the film. Okay, I told myself, it's a new year and a new me. Be gone, pneumonia. I'm off to make a movie.

Reluctantly, I gave up coproducing the film in favor of starring in it with Charlie. Shaking off the remnants of my illness, I left for Washington, D.C., and location filming. On the first day, while awaiting a shot, I tipped my chair backward against a wall for support. I was pleased with my First Lady image, swaddled in a black mink coat from the wardrobe department, when suddenly I was deluged with cold coffee.

In an upper story of the building someone, cleaning offices, dumped all the coffee urns out of a window. My hair, mink coat, and stylish shoes were saturated. I looked up only to receive another urnful in the face. So much for the glamorous movie life. Not my first such experience.

It reminded me of the previous year in London on location with Charlie. I had bought myself a new black-linen suit to wear at lunch with Charlie and director Michael Winner. I stepped out of the car, smoothed my skirt to make an elegant appearance, when suddenly from overhead it seemed as if someone had emptied a bucket of whitewash. Splash! My hair and suit were covered in white and green. It was not whitewash. I discovered it was the work of an extraordinarily large pigeon.

Charlie saw me coming toward him, grumbling and wiping. I explained.

"That's lucky, baby," Charlie said, laughing. "Anyway, I hate that suit; you know I don't like your shoulders to be bigger than mine."

Now I had two baptisms to prove that pride often *does* go before a fall.

42

Jill's House

1986

The proceeds of my participation in *My Affair with the President's Wife*—later retitled *Assassination*—helped to buy a beach cottage in Malibu. Cassie, my devoted German shepherd, and I enjoy it most because we're beach creatures.

The house sits directly on the beach. Two bedrooms, an L-shaped sitting room, and a small kitchen. The sound and tang of the sea engulf me. The veranda overlooks the beach, and huge, jagged, primeval rocks, dark brown and filled with tide pools and crustaceans, jut from a bed of kelp.

I have finally found a place that gives me peace of mind. The ocean is always restless and I love the incessant conversation it holds with the shore.

Charlie and I also bought another house at Serra in Malibu that would become our main family residence. I never imagined I would be the mistress of two homes within three miles of each other, but this is precisely the case. It takes only three minutes for me to drive from our Serra home to my cottage.

"Think of it, Charlie," I said, hoping he would love the

little beach cottage the way I had learned to love Vermont, "now when we want a holiday, we can simply jump in the car or even walk to our vacation house."

Charlie looked enigmatic. We now had two homes in Malibu, one in Bel Air, and one in Vermont. So much for simplification.

43

The Torch Bearer

1986

In the summer I received a telephone call from my mother. She was desperately tired from taking care of her husband and dealing with the death of her sister Edith. Mummy was stricken with a painful case of shingles. It was clear she was completely exhausted and needed nurturing.

It was decided my sister-in-law Sandra would fly to England to stay at my parents' bungalow and take care of my truculent father while Mummy visited me and Charlie at the beach house. The small cottage folded loving, protective arms around her and I was able to watch Mummy's strength return.

But looking after Jack proved no simple task for Sandra.

Sandra calls him Jack and thinks he's cute. My father also thinks he is pretty cute and is quite accustomed to managing the women in his life, ruling the roost of his attractive little home. But Jack and Sandra could not anticipate the events of the three weeks they shared.

Sandra arrived prepared to play the happy little housewife, washing out her smalls and hanging them on the line.

She later told me, "I'm glad I brought my best underwear. I was embarrassed seeing my panties and bras flapping on the wash line in the garden for anyone to see. But I feel like such a good little housewife. And Jack's being a sweetheart."

The honeymoon was brief.

During one phone call between Malibu and Seaford, Sandra said, "Your father's looking rather stern and he's glancing at the clock."

"He thinks you're on the phone too long," I suggested.

"It's okay, Jack," she said to him. "Jill doesn't mind."

"Hmmm," said Jack, pointing at the clock. "Lo lo lo."

"Put him on the line," I said.

"Lo lo lo," said my father in a growly tone.

"It's okay, Daddy. Let Sandra use the phone. She needs to talk to me. Now, don't be an old meanie. And don't give her any trouble."

"Lo lo lo," said a definitely disgruntled Jack, who walked away leaving the phone dangling.

Sandra laughed merrily. "Oh, he's so cute, but he's being quite surly now."

"He growls when Mummy and I talk too long," I told her. "He knows I'm paying for the call but he doesn't want me to spend my money. It's one of his ways of controlling things. You know how he likes to be master of all he surveys."

"I'm beginning to see it more clearly every day."

"Lo lo lo," came from the background, ever more growly.

"Now, Jack," Sandra said. "Don't do that. It's very rude."

Then *click*; that's all I heard. I knew Jack had taken the phone from her hand and hung up.

A few minutes passed and the telephone rang.

"Jill, I had to go round to the neighbor's house. Your father's being absolutely impossible. He's an old tyrant. Every time I go near the phone he brandishes his cane at me and says 'lo lo lo.' So I told him, 'I won't stand for this,' and I walked out of the house."

The next day Sandra called again. "He's out on his walk. He won't know about this call. When I returned yesterday he was quite abashed and sitting quietly in his chair. He probably thought I'd taken a walk, but we tricked him, didn't we?"

"Yes," I agreed, "but you better not let him catch you calling from the neighbors'."

The following day I spoke to my father, who was quite pleasant until Sandra took the line. The *lo lo los* began again in the background.

"Don't you speak to me like that, Jack," Sandra said, stamping her foot.

"Oh. Lo lo?" said my father in an inquiring tone, obviously asking, "What's this then? Is this you putting your foot down, Sandra?"

"I won't have it, Jack," said Sandra firmly.

"Let him have it," I said from my safe seat across the ocean.

Click!

Jack had obviously taken matters into his own hand again.

Minutes later Sandra was calling from the neighbors'. "Jill, he's absolutely impossible. He just walks over me. He takes the phone right out of my hand. I can't have a wrestling match with the old man. I don't know how your mother handles it. Their neighbor, a very nice lady, tells me when your father flies off the handle, the whole street can hear him. Nobody knows how your mother manages him.

"Something must be done," Sandra went on. "Your mother's trip to Malibu is like sticking on a Band-Aid. She'll come back and he will wear her down again. He's exhausting, demanding, and a creature of habit. Everything has to happen at the same time every day—his breakfast, his walk, his lunch at exactly the same time. If not he *'lo lo los'* and taps on the clock. How does your mother handle it?"

I said, "I suppose that's why she's ill. Poor Mummy. She's like a puppet and he's pulling the strings. We'll have to do something."

We agreed my parents wanted to keep their home and Sandra suggested that my mother put Jack in a nursing home one week in every four to ensure herself a week of rest every month.

I agreed, saying, "Mother is so exhausted she seems to have given up. Actually, she brought one or two pieces of good silver, things she wanted to give me 'in case anything happens.' She should have some quality time. I don't know if she will agree to sending Daddy to a home because he hates those places."

Sandra convinced me the nursing home where Daddy had been placed when Mummy became ill was lovely and right on the sea. She had picked him up at the home on her arrival in Seaford.

"The place is called Three Ways and the rooms are very nice with TV sets, and the staff seemed fond of him," she said. "It's not like anything you'd imagine for an old-age home. It's a place to convalesce, and they love Jack there. Except, did you hear, Jill, he got into a fight with an old man?"

"My God, no. When?"

Sandra laughed. "It happened when your mother dropped him off. It was the talk of the place. There was another cantankerous gentleman whom everyone disliked. He evidently offended your father by suggesting he was an idiot because he couldn't speak. Jack punched him on the nose with his one good arm. The doctor told me he was glad Jack did it. He said the old man had it coming; everyone wanted to punch him on the nose."

When I stopped laughing at the prospect of a fistfight in

a convalescent home, Sandra said, "It's not easy to cross Jack."

She added another, more touching story. A distinguished judge was admitted to the nursing home after suffering a massive stroke that left him partially paralyzed and unable to speak. He was frightened and confused. My father found him alone in a corner and sat beside him. The nurses said it was a moving sight to see the two aphasia victims exchanging gibberish. Daddy obviously tried to reassure the man as best he could with his *lo lo* intonations. Gradually, the judge's fright diminished. He was not alone. He took comfort in the knowledge that at least one other resident of the home had suffered the same dreadful tragedy and knew what he was going through. My father was sorrowful and kept giving the man sad looks. When he caught his eye, he smiled as if saying, "Don't worry; you'll be all right."

Less than twenty-four hours later, Sandra was back on the telephone. "Do you know what that old bugger did today?"

I quickly called mother to pick up an extension.

"You know your mother put a new jet in the fireplace to avoid building a coal fire every day," Sandra went on. "She told me Jack was never allowed to light the fire by himself because with one hand he can't strike a match."

My mother spoke up. "Yes, Sandra, I know. Of course he's not supposed to do it."

"Well, I got up early this morning but Jack was up even earlier. I walked from the bedroom to the sitting room and *whoomp!*—a huge bang and suddenly black everywhere. I nearly had a heart attack."

"Oh, no," said my mother. "He didn't."

"Yes, he did," said Sandra. "He'd lit the fire. And do you know how, Dorothy?"

"Yes," my mother said in a weak voice. "He turns up the gas jet, then gets a newspaper, rolls it up, lights the newspaper from the pilot light on the kitchen stove, and runs through the house."

"Exactly. Like an Olympic torch carrier," Sandra said.

Mother added, "He runs through the house carrying the Olympic flame . . ."

". . . through a gas-filled room," Sandra interjected.

"My God. Then what?" I wanted to know.

"By the time he gets to the fireplace the room is full of gas, but he sticks the torch into the fireplace and *whoomp!* It's bad enough we risk our lives, but the whole place is black."

"Have you cleaned it up?" my mother asked.

"Yes," Sandra replied irritably. "But my nerves are still shaking. When I told him never to do it again, Jack was meek and quite crestfallen. He went to his room, changed, and disappeared on a walk. That's why I'm calling. We've still got black on the ceiling, Dorothy."

Now I was laughing. I could see my old man running sneakily through the sitting room in his shorts each morning so Sandra would not see his Olympic act.

"Sandra, you poor thing," I said.

"He's so cute and funny," she said. "We had a flaming row the other day and I stamped my foot at him and he said, 'Oooh.' He usually doesn't make those noises, then he covered his mouth with his hand and giggled. It was as if he were saying, 'Feisty little thing, isn't she?'

"He put his arm around me and tried to give me a kiss on the cheek. I was furious so I said, 'No good, Jack.' I went to my room and slammed the door and called through it, 'I want to be alone awhile, Jack; I don't want to see you.' Ten minutes went by and suddenly Jack was back with a bar of chocolate and a whiskey."

My mother said, "He always did think that was the way to a woman's heart."

By now I was roaring with laughter, which irritated

Sandra and my mother because they could not hear one another.

Sandra continued. "He gave me the whiskey and the chocolate, then put his hand on one side of his face with that cute look of his . . ."

"Yes, yes," said my mother, "he always does that, and a sweet smile?"

"And one of the sweetest smiles you've ever seen. Then he said, 'Lo lo' in a quiet voice, 'lo lo, lo?' I told him, 'All right, Jack . . .'"

"Did you eat the chocolate?" I asked.

"Of course I ate the chocolate, what do you think I am? A fool? Then I drank the whiskey and I felt much better. Afterward I sat with Jack and made him promise he would behave. And what do I find this morning?"

"*Whoomp*," said my mother.

"Exactly," Sandra said. "Oh, oh, he's coming, I'd better hang up."

"He's still manipulating you, Sandra," I said.

"You're damn right. I'm going to stay on the phone."

There was a hesitation, then Sandra spoke again, "Hello, Jack, would you like to speak to your wife? I told them what you did this morning."

"Oh, lo lo lo," said a low, mournful voice.

"Come on, she wants to speak to you. So does Jill."

With a clattering and clanking he picked up the phone. "Lo lo lo," my father said in a deeper tone.

"Lo lo, yourself," I said. "You're trying to kill yourself and Sandra in the bargain."

"Jack," said my mother, "you know you're never to light the fire. You know you can't do it."

"Lo lo lo."

"Daddy, you should be shot. Sandra's in a terrible state. And don't you think whiskey and chocolate will do it this time. You better have a word with her."

"Lo lo," he said hopefully, thinking, yes, I probably can manage it. She's only a woman after all.

"And, Daddy, don't dare try to light the fire again."

"Don't do it, Jack," my mother chorused.

"Lo lo," said my father perkily. "Lo lo." And then he hung up.

"God," I said, "now Sandra's lost another chance to have the last word."

"That's the way he is, Jill," Dorothy said. "We'll never change him."

Later that day my mother sat on the beach-house veranda looking around for Henry Isaacs, a gentleman of uncertain age. The previous evening Mother, for the first time, dressed herself up, declared her shingles almost gone, and joined me at my neighbor Cynthia Lindsay's house for drinks. We were given two extra-large vodka and tonics by Robert Patten, Cynthia's longtime love. My mother drank hers and was immediately given another.

While I made polite conversation with two ladies, I heard my mother say, "Well, I would, Henry, dear, but it's my party piece."

"Oh, go ahead, Dorothy, do," I heard.

My mother looked at me questioningly.

"Why not, Mother? Do it, whatever it is. Give it a rip." Dorothy set out:

All the nice girls love a sailor
All the nice girls love a tar.
There's something about a sailor,
And you know what sailors are.

My mother sang this coyly in a rather vaudevillian way.

"It's my party piece," she said at the end. "That's as much as I do. And I think, Jill, we'd better try to make an exit gracefully while we still can."

"I won't tell Daddy."

Henry Isaacs was appalled. "You mean there's a *Mr.* Ireland?"

My mother said rather sheepishly, "Oh, yes."

"But you didn't tell me. You've been leading me along," he said.

I smiled to myself. When I first walked in I had seen Henry and said, "I was always nice to your mother, Henry, now it's up to you to be nice to mine."

Clearly, Henry had taken me literally and was flirting the old girl's legs off.

"I'll look out for you tomorrow, Dorothy," he said. "I'm staying over tonight."

"She'll be on the veranda in the morning in her swimsuit," I said.

"No, I won't, Jill," said Mummy.

"Yes, you will," I replied taking my mother home where she slept sweetly and, I hope, had pleasant dreams.

But now she was standing on the veranda in her swimsuit sunning her toes, Cassie at her side.

"I think it's doing your father good," she said, "having someone else staying at home with him."

"I'm sure it's opening Sandra's eyes, too," I added.

I sat on the porch beside my mother, controlling my desire to laugh aloud as a picture floated in my mind of a blizzard of black ashes floating down on my parents' cheery sitting room, and my father, like a marathon runner on his last legs, underwear drooping, as barefoot he made his way across the gas-filled room, saying, "Oh, boy, I got away with it this time."

I could not help but imagine, somewhere in England, my triumphant father warming his shanks and his one good hand before the satisfying blaze that he had created while Sandra, like Cinderella, swept up cinders and mopped up the soot.

After three weeks my mother became homesick for her little house and her husband, so she packed her small bag, donned her traveling suit, had a shampoo, set, and manicure at the local beauty shop, and took the overnight flight from Los Angeles to London full of anticipation at showing off her California suntan. In her suitcase, wrapped in silver paper and carefully padded amongst her underthings, she packed two ripe avocados as a treat for my father.

44

Mother's Birthday

1986

One day I telephoned my mother and from the sound of her voice I knew that something was wrong. All the relaxation was gone from her tone. The term *shattered* entered my mind as I listened to those first few words.

"Hello, Jill. I wondered if it was you."

I was calling to wish her happy birthday. Due to the time difference it was eight in the evening in England. Instead of happiness, which I had wished for her on her eightieth birthday, I could tell she had been weeping.

Reluctantly, she told me how my father in a fit of frustrated rage raised his fists high above his head and then brought them down accidentally, as she put it, and struck her.

"He hit me, Jill. I couldn't understand something he wanted. He kept badgering me. I know it was an accident, but he hit me on the chest and I nearly fainted."

I said in some alarm, "Can he raise both his arms when he's angry, Mother?"

"Oh, yes, he raises both, even the paralyzed one. And he

shouts gibberish at me. Screams it. I'm sure everybody in the whole street can hear him. I just stand in front of him and I don't move. I don't dare move because I think if I do that arm will come down.

"And this time he did it. I had just cooked a wonderful dinner for Daddy and me. It is my birthday, you see, Jill. I cooked a roast beef and Yorkshire pudding. And I'd made myself a little birthday cake. You know these days I don't cook so much. I get too tired. It's hard enough taking care of your father without cooking special dinners in the evening. But this was my birthday. Eighty. I'd just put it on the table and then, I don't know why, because as you know I can't understand a word he says, your father suddenly lost his temper. It spoiled my dinner, but I sat down and ate it anyway."

"Oh, Mummy, I'm so sorry. You deserve the most wonderful birthday. It's so unfair. When Daddy turned eighty he had such a lovely day with friends visiting, gifts, and telephone calls. People made a fuss of him all day."

At this point my mother broke into tears.

"I didn't want you to know, Jill. I never wanted you to know."

"But I knew, Mummy. I've always known. We all have."

"I do feel better now I've shared it," she said.

"Well, Mummy, you tell me any time you feel the need. Let me talk to Daddy. I'll tell him he mustn't do it."

"Oh, no, don't talk to him now. It might make him angry again. I feel ever so much better for talking to you. I love you, Jill."

"I love you too, Mummy."

I hung up the telephone and, wanting to be alone, I sat on the porch steps of the beach house facing the ocean, listening to the healing waves, watching them break over the big rock, visualizing my brain as that rock. I tried to feel the water washing clean all the fragments of thoughts and painful feelings. I wrote a letter to my father.

Dear Daddy:

Before I write another word, I must preface this letter with I love you. I have the greatest admiration for you. You are my inspiration, your courage, strength, and determination in the face of your terrible handicap, a handicap you received as the direct result of my urging open-heart surgery. So you see, I carry a burden of guilt—the guilt of interfering with your life out of a selfish childish need to have you around a bit longer.

You see, Daddy, as I was growing up, I didn't really get to know you. Then when I was in my late thirties, when you had your surgery, and I was a mother myself, I still needed my daddy. So I overrode your insistence that you had enough strength when you were saying, "I think I'm all right, Jill. I think I have enough strength to go on as long as I'm supposed to."

I talked you out of your own instinctive knowledge so hard won after your many illnesses and painful surgeries. Yes, I remember your vow after the last operation never to go under the surgeon's knife again. But I used all the power of my persuasion to get you to let them open your chest and replace five of the valves to your brave heart.

Oh, Daddy, was I wrong? My father, whom I hardly knew, the man who now cannot speak to me of his feelings and frustrations. I love you, Daddy. But this I must write also.

Don't bully my mother anymore. Don't shout at her. She is old, Daddy; she does her best. She has been such a good and loyal wife. I know that her ambitions in many ways didn't match yours. She wouldn't uproot her family and go to Australia when as a younger man you so desired a new start. But, Daddy, she has spent a decade tending to you so stoically, matching your valor as you both, reeling from the shock of the never-ending reality of your devastating stroke, lived on together through your seventies, a decade of living, never again to have a proper conversation, never a joke or a remark.

It's hard for her too. And I know she shares your pain and frustration. So please don't give her the full content of your rage, your sorrow, your hatred of your fate. It's not her fault. And in her old age she cannot go on with the stress that you give her. She wants to, but she's faltering. She needs help.

Daddy, you must not rage at her again. You will destroy her and, in doing so, destroy yourself. I don't know what you can do when the feelings in you rise, threatening to choke you, when your tears don't fall but instead burn and scorch your soul. You don't deserve this fate.

Charlie said to me, "I'm afraid we did the wrong thing." I cried because we are responsible for the unending prison of life into which we've locked you, a life without the ability to communicate with another soul by speaking or writing.

My heart breaks for you but also for my indefatigably loyal mother. So please don't use her as an emotional dumping ground. Please. I have no answers, no cures. We are all locked in. I only know she shouldn't be bullied and intimidated and sad in these last years of her life.

I did not send this letter because two days after my mother's birthday, my father suffered another small stroke.

45
Confrontation

1986

Charlie's relationship with Jason was supercharged with emotion. Love, anger, frustration, and pride, like electric currents, crackled between these two vastly different males.

By turns Charlie was compassionate and generous, then suspicious, resentful, and furious toward my adopted son. Charlie was the real father figure in Jason's life, and from the first Jason had loved this strong, silent man with a dogged determination. The more Jason strove to please Charlie, the farther he seemed to be pushed away.

It appeared as if Jason's enthusiasm overwhelmed Charlie's sensibilities. Their ongoing relationship brings to mind a large exuberant dog lovingly leaping up on its master with muddy paws, seeking approbation, attention, and love. The recipient of this mixed blessing of affection and annoyance tends to step back, pleased by the display of devotion but repelled by the disquieting results. Despite his good intentions, Jason always seemed to defeat his own purpose in his attempts to demonstrate his love for Charlie.

As I prepared for my coming book tour it should have been the best time in my life. The book had been well received; the reviews were, happily, uniformly good and encouraging.

A few days before the tour, I was in my dressing room sorting through outfits to take along. Jason had been in the master bedroom talking to Charlie. He was obviously depressed as he passed my door. I saw his tall, stiff walk. His legs were clearly hurting. I thought immediately he was back on drugs.

Why hadn't I seen it sooner? The signs were all there. Jason's eyes were full of pain when we talked. There was a white, almost greenish tinge to his skin. He perspired constantly. He was out of work and in debt. A whine returned to his voice and he was always in a hurry. This morning it was a most unhappy man who responded to my call.

"Come and sit down, Jason. What's going on?"

"Oh, I was trying to discuss something with Charlie. But he doesn't want to talk right now."

He paced the floor, full of tension. "I think about my real father. Would he sit down with me and listen? Would he talk to me?"

"Jason, would you like to find your father?"

My son looked at me. "No, I was just the outcome of a one-night stand. I'd just find more trouble."

"Please, sit down beside me."

"No, I can't, Mom; I've got to keep walking. I hurt."

The room filled with sadness. Here I was again, confronting Jason. As I beheld his thin body, looking into his drawn face, I saw the magical dark-blue eyes now huge and desperate. He was talking about Charlie.

"It's stand up, sit down, again. I don't need this."

The day had started with such optimism. It was to be a good, productive day, discussing Zuleika Farm deals with Sue Overholt. Then a newspaper interview followed by a television interview. I felt the tears start.

Jason said, "Mom, don't cry; bastards like me survive. People like you take all the shit and hurt. You're good, Mom; you don't deserve this."

Jason departed like a wraith. Earlier in the morning I had thought about washing my hair and getting myself ready for the television interview in a leisurely way. Yes, the day *had* been full of promise; but ten minutes with Jason and I was tense and heartbroken.

I went downstairs to the bar and swallowed two big gulps of Courvoisier brandy to steady myself. A TV crew was coming up to the house to interview me, the got-it-together lady who had beaten cancer.

I recalled Jason telling me I was good. I didn't think so. Only that morning Charlie had called me a nag, manipulative and bossy; and I knew I probably was. I know I try to control things around the people I love.

Was *I* the problem?

No, I couldn't take that responsibility.

At midday Jason came into the sitting room to find me at my desk.

"Mom." His face was haggard. "Call Larry [Martindale, our business manager]. I have to pay my Nippers bill."

"I told you to bring all your bills to me," I said, remembering Nippers was a nightclub Jason frequented.

"I'm sorry." His voice took on an agonizing defensive tone. "I made a mistake."

At this moment Charlie came in and immediately he and Jason were engaged in a verbal battle that could have no victor. I had tried to avoid a confrontation between these two men by paying Jason's Nippers bill before it came to Charlie's attention. Unfortunately, Jason had erred in sending the bill to Larry Martindale and it ended up on Charlie's desk. Now what I had most feared happened.

They went upstairs and I was worried, knowing how fragile Jason was. Through the ceiling, as I sat at my desk, I could hear the male voices raised in anger. And then, to my horror, I heard banging and thumping. A fight was going on. I forced myself to sit still and not do what I had done so many times before—get into the middle of the fight.

It would be less than an hour before the TV crew arrived. My eyes were still swollen from crying. Suddenly there was silence and I feared the worst.

Jason came down, looked at me, and showed me a watch and three-hundred dollars in cash.

"There you are," he said cockily, his self-esteem momentarily restored. "Charlie gave me this and the money to pay my bills."

My heart sank when I saw the cash in my son's hand, and as for the watch, it was a twenty-dollar copy of the Cartier tank watch, which Charlie had picked up on a movie set. Jason thought it was genuine, and I have no idea why Charlie gave it to him except as a peace offering. I wondered how I could pull myself together to do the TV show.

I felt abused. I had gone to bat for Jason by trying to pay his bills. I had sat silently while I thought a murder was taking place upstairs. And now here he was with a cheap watch and cash. Money in the hand of an addict is like razor blades in the hand of a monkey. There would be no bills paid this day. I was furious.

"Damn it, Jason, why didn't you just give the bills to me?"

I felt my frustration rising.

Jason went to his bedroom. I knew communication was hopeless but I would try once more. To my surprise and embarrassment, I found his young glamour-girlfriend Sabina in his bed, her round, cheerful face wreathed in a smile. Jason was drinking a beer.

I took the beer can from his hand and threw it at him, enraged. I was in turmoil physically and emotionally and he was playing it cool.

Jason went berserk. We fought. I hit him and then grabbed him as he tried to leave the room. I threw a bed-frame that for some reason had been propped against a wall. It struck him a glancing blow. Jason fled and I ran up the stairs on his heels.

He was shouting that I was crazy and threatened to sue me, just as he had threatened whenever, as a child, he had been angry with someone.

I stopped and could do nothing but weep hopeless tears. All I could see was my son with no sense of reality.

I returned to his room to apologize to the girl. I told Sabina I was totally unprepared to find someone in Jason's room, and that I was angry to find a stranger in my house. The girl was sympathetic. She got out of bed immediately and put her arms around me.

"It's all right," she said, "it's all right," which made me cry harder.

"I'm sorry I threw the beer," I said.

The TV crew was due shortly.

It was too late to wash my hair, so I simply fluffed it up with styling gel, put on a pink angora sweater, and somehow managed to immerse myself in the question-and-answer session for the nationally syndicated show.

How the hell could I help anyone else when I couldn't even get my mascara on straight because my hands were shaking? Somehow I got dressed and made up. I did not look my best, to be sure, but once I sat in the big antique chair in the sitting room and faced the cameras and the subject of cancer and how I cope with it, I was on familiar terrain. How ironic, I could fight my own enemy within, but I could not fight the enemy without, Jason's enemy— drug addiction.

Oh, I seemed so on top of it all. I had it made. The beautiful home, the celebrated husband, a book published and headed for the best-seller list and a movie out; all in the same month.

The next day my mother called with bad news. It was not yet enough that Jason was on drugs again. Mummy told me Daddy had had another stroke, albeit a small one. Now his tongue seemed paralyzed. No more *lo lo lo* for him. His mouth was twisted and all he could utter was *ah ah ah* in a weak, downward-sounding pattern. Daddy had never been affectionately demonstrative after the brief period of my toddler years. In fact, I never heard my father say *I love you*. Now, when I sensed so strongly that he wanted to say those words, all he could utter was *ah ah ah*.

Dear God, was I going to watch my father die in bits and pieces as Jason died slowly from drugs and alcohol? I could not ignore either situation. I could never stop watching by turning the proverbial blind eye.

I took my dog Cassie for a long walk around UCLA's beautiful campus. The walk helped. Tears burned my eyes and cheeks, but I calmed down after an hour. I came home, took a shower, and felt physically better. I hoped I would handle the stress more easily the next time around. I had to. I had offered myself up as light at the end of the tunnel, hadn't I?

Jason came through the door of the Bel Air house in late afternoon with Sabina. I was gladdened by the sight of him, although he looked more thin and gaunt than ever.

"Happy birthday, darling," I said, giving him a hug. A flicker of fear rippled somewhere in my brain.

Jason was smiling, but something else was there.

Now fear spread to my stomach and between my ribs. I could no longer deny the signs.

I asked him to step on the scales. He weighed only one hundred twenty-six pounds in his trousers and shoes. I saw every bone in his rib cage; his arms and legs were stick thin. He restlessly complained of cramps in his legs and back. He cracked his neck constantly to ease the discomfort.

I had arranged dinner at home, but only Val and Katrina were there for the celebration. Charlie was working late and everyone else had lost faith in Jason's turning up at all for his birthday dinner. He wanted to go out to dinner, saying, "I want lobster, Mom."

Happy to indulge him, I booked reservations for Val, Katrina, Jason, Sabina, and myself at an Italian restaurant where we had played so many scenes in the past. I booked the table for seven o'clock, but at six-forty-five Jason was not ready to go. He wandered restlessly around the house.

"You go ahead, Mom; I'll meet you there."

Val, Katrina, and I waited at the restaurant for twenty minutes before a harassed-looking Jason arrived with Sabina. He ordered dinner and a vodka and grapefruit juice. But when the lobster arrived, Jason wouldn't eat. He showed me some sores on the inside of his mouth. He complained they burned so much he was unable to sip his drink. The tender areas of his mouth reminded me of the sores I had had when I was undergoing chemotherapy.

While we were occupied with dinner, Jason left the table to make a lengthy telephone call. He walked to and from the men's room and the bar before joining us again.

"Mom, do you have forty bucks?"

"Why?" I asked, losing heart. I was tired of fighting my son. I was tired of withholding money that I thought would go for drugs.

"Here, Jason," I said, opening my wallet. I couldn't really help or talk to him, but I could give him money. It was almost a relief to be able to do something for him, no matter what.

"I need to get some pot," he explained. "It will relax me, and then I'll be able to eat."

He went off again to the telephone.

Somewhere inside me I had made a decision. I couldn't stop this person from taking drugs. I loved him so much I decided to buy them for him, as many drugs as he needed until he stopped. I rationalized that on his birthday the only significant gift I could give him was drugs, the single present he truly wanted or needed on this special day. It dawned on me that I had reached a devastating level myself, willing to feed my son's drug habit in order to assure him of my love.

The four of us ate our dinners in dismal silence while Jason's plate remained untouched. Katrina took her fork and pronged a bit of his lobster.

I became possessive. "Don't, Katrina," I snapped, "it's Jason's food."

The waiter packed it in a container, along with some chocolate mousse that Jason would eat later at home after he had made contact with someone who would sell him forty dollars' worth of grass.

I was hoping his dealer would be home. God! What had I come to?

At home in bed I admitted to myself that Jason was on cocaine again. I wept myself to sleep only to awaken at five in the morning to go downstairs to see if he were there. He was. I had asked him not to have drugs delivered to our home.

"God, Mom, you don't know how much stuff has been delivered to this house."

I knew it was true. I felt soiled. It was a nightmare. People like Kadafi, the small Asian who had been to the house a couple of times, were obviously suppliers. How could I change all this? I could do nothing except perhaps get Jason an apartment and let him kill himself.

After all, I had my other children to think about, Zuleika in particular. I believed Jason could not survive long on his own. But could I survive living with him?

In a day or two I would be on the road, a traveling dog-and-pony show talking about *Life Wish*. The words of the title mocked me.

46
Book Tour

1987

I embarked on a fourteen-stop tour of the major American cities, including New York, and branching out from city to city to appear on TV and radio talk shows.

It began on a curious note. I appeared on Joan Rivers's Los Angeles late-night talk show, which was taped in the evening. Immediately thereafter I boarded a plane for San Francisco with Sue Overholt and my publicist Lori Jonas. We arrived at San Francisco Airport where we passed a taproom in which a TV set was surrounded by a large group of men engrossed in watching an athletic event.

Lori barged in, dragging Sue and me behind her. She strode to the set and switched channels to watch Joan's show to see how I had performed. The moment she touched the set a howl of protest went up from the men who continued to growl and grumble at the nerve of this tiny female who had cut off their entertainment. I tried to be inconspicuous, terrified lest any of the crowd identify me as the source of their anger. Fortunately, they did not and Lori declared herself pleased with the show.

The tour was a jumble of airports, limousine rides through cities that looked alike from the car, then hotel lobbies, broadcasting studios, smiling talk-show hosts, and meals from room service in impersonal hotel rooms—New York, Detroit, Philadelphia, Cleveland, St. Louis, Minneapolis, Rochester, Toronto. They all ran together. It was a pity I had no time to see the beauty and individuality of America's great urban centers.

I remember one flight from New York to Detroit, after Lori had returned to her business activities in Los Angeles. I wore a white-cotton sweatsuit and Reeboks and was reading a book about Charles Manson. I looked out at a flame-red skyline, dramatically layered between gray clouds and soft shades of turquoise blue sky blending into the ink-black night above.

I saw what appeared to be black smoke tendriling upward from the clouds, slowly blotting out the orange-flame remnants of the sunset. Charles Manson and an ominous skyline, hardly the sort of inspiration I should harbor.

Jill Ireland, what are you doing? Role playing? I searched my conscience while the sky turned darker, daring me to fool myself. Why was I touring? Really. I wasn't fooling myself. I truly wanted to talk to people who, like me, were playing out the rest of their lives on the gift of borrowed time, we ex-cancer patients. How could I even for a moment doubt my intentions?

I was not a glory seeker, but it was difficult to ignore the compliments, admiration, and affection that came my way on the tour.

"I want to thank you for writing the book," was an oft-repeated phrase. *Inspirational, courageous, brave* were used to describe me, but I didn't feel brave. I began to feel as if I were unsuspectingly giving suck to a baby tiger that I would soon hold by the tail. I would not become a professional cancer victim.

I was going out there to make brave little speeches about fighting for my life while my own son was unable to come to grips with his. There was a heavy, dead feeling inside. Jason, why can't I inspire and help you? You whom I love so dearly? I have used all my intellect, all my emotions. I have searched my soul for the words, the love, the means to convince you to fight for your life. My God, Jason, where have you gone? Little boy, give me another chance. Come back to me. Wasn't my love enough?

I sensed—indeed I knew—Jason was in some sort of trouble while I was on tour. Charlie's evasive answers on the telephone were a sure indication. Hardly a moment passed during my sweep of the country when I wasn't concerned about my son.

My love for Jason, I'm sure, is blazingly clear. But that does not mean I love Paul, Valentine, and Zuleika less, or even my stepchildren and my adopted daughter Katrina. I love them all, but love comes in different forms and intensities. My love for my two Englishmen, Valentine and Paul, is singular.

Valentine is special to me. From the time he was a baby, he gave me much pleasure. He was the most cuddly, sensitive child, full of love, and he still is. Valentine tends to be a bit of a baffled professor much of the time. He's highly intelligent and dedicated to his work as a composer-musician. On the other hand, he tends to lose sweaters, keys, books, telephone numbers, etc. No amount of coaxing helps. My hope is one day he will marry a warm, sexy, responsible woman who will keep his life intact while he goes about the serious business of his work. Valentine is generous; he would give you the shirt off his back if he could remember where he put it.

My youngest son is also placid. One night I returned home to find his pickup truck blocking the entrance to my garage, a transgression about which he had been warned many times. In a fury, I leaped from my car and kicked in the door on the driver's side of his truck, leaving an enormous dent. When I dragged Valentine from the house to show him what I'd done by way of punishment, a look of bemusement suffused his handsome face. My six-foot-six-inch giant moved his truck to its proper parking space and ambled back into the house without a word.

On another evening, when Zuleika was a scant fourteen, I entrusted her to the care of Valentine and Katrina who were taking her to a party attended by their friends. When the trio returned home, my little Zuleika was staggeringly tipsy. Someone at the party had given her a drink.

I calmly took her upstairs to her bedroom, undressed her, and put her to bed. Before I could remonstrate, she said drunkenly. "Oh, Mother, will you ever forgive me? I'm *very* young." Then she slipped away into a peaceful sleep.

I came out of Zuleika's room shaken and angry. I looked at Val: "How dare you bring your sister home like this?

"And you, Katrina," I said, pointing a finger, "stop crying."

Val attempted to leave the sitting room, somewhat on his high horse.

I said, "Val, sit down."

He sat in the nearest chair, which brought him to the right height for me to sock him on the jaw.

He took it like a man.

"That's for bringing your sister home drunk," I said, as I massaged my swollen and sore knuckles.

It didn't help my fury to note that while my hand was red and painful, Val's face showed nary a mark. To make matters worse, there was a suspicion of a smile at the corners of his mouth, which he was obviously trying to control.

Both my Englishmen tend to be amused when *their little mother* becomes enraged. They are never terrified.

Val said nothing, taking my cuffing almost as a matter of course. When I demanded an answer, he said, "I'm sorry, Mom. It will never happen again."

And, of course, it never did.

My relationship with Katrina, now on the eve of her twenties, continues to deepen and give me great joy. We behave as woman-to-woman, more so day by day. There is nothing we can't discuss. She is a passionate, intelligent girl.

Sometimes I felt guilty about the amount of time and money I devoted to Jason, perhaps at the expense of my other children. I spent a fortune on Jason's rehabilitation, detoxing and hospitalization.

My concern encouraged me to talk to Val. One evening we were in the sitting room and I said, "Val, I love you very much. I know Jason takes a lot of attention. Charlie has accused me of favoring Jason. This just isn't true. I don't favor anyone over you. You're my funny Valentine, my sweet Valentine."

My good, strong young man who had never been a problem since his birth, enfolded me in his arms.

I said, "You know what they say about the squeaky wheel getting the oil, and Jason has been squeaking since birth."

"I know, Mom. I understand. I love Jason, too. And I'm going to help him one day. I could teach him the studio sound board. I could . . ."

I stopped him. "Val, I don't want Jason to become your responsibility. Please remember, if anything ever happens to me, don't make Jason your responsibility. I know you love him. You're almost like twins. You can't remember life without Jason, but do not let his drug addiction ruin your life."

Paul was as reliable as Valentine and considerably more independent. My eldest Englishman had been living in his own apartment for many years. At twenty-nine he is prospering with his karate and scuba teaching and music composition.

I promised myself there would be gifts for both my Englishmen before my money drained entirely into the deep hole Jason had dug with needles, cocaine spoons, and reefer wrappings. After all, my nest egg came from the sale of the Hollywood home David and I had bought. It was money from myself and the father of my sons; the proceeds rightfully belonged to the Englishmen.

Both Paul and Val wanted to help Jason, and I had leaned heavily on Paul for moral support many times. But I told him, as I had Val, "Break loose. Jason's not your responsibility."

That was easier said than done. We all loved Jason. We were the original McCallum group, me, Jason, and Val, and in David's absence Paul was surrogate father to his younger brothers.

I snapped out of my reverie as the airplane circled and I could see Detroit spread out beneath me. I was back to reality. Sue would locate the ten pieces of luggage, find a limousine, and get us to the hotel in time for eight hours' sleep. It had been many days since I had enjoyed that luxury.

Several days later Sue and I arrived in Montreal. I was tired and running on empty and looking forward to an hour to myself before going on TV. We would go directly to our hotel, order a meal, take a bath, get made up, and then go to the studio. But the plane was late and our luggage lost.

I was horrified. I had made the trip in a black jumpsuit, wearing no makeup and with not a scrap of makeup in my handbag. How could I go on TV in a jumpsuit and without makeup?

While Sue looked for our luggage I lay down on the nearest counter. Passersby stared in astonishment as they saw me lying supine, pale, dressed in black, and my head resting on my handbag.

We were supposed to be met by one of the local TV representatives. Two rather distinguished-looking gentlemen gave me a cursory look and went on to greener pastures. I obviously wasn't what they were expecting. Sue learned our bags had been placed on another plane and would be joining us in two hours, too late for the TV performance. As she informed me of this, the distinguished-looking gentlemen returned and tentatively approached me.

"Are you . . ."

". . . Jill Ireland?" I said.

They chorused, "Yes."

"That's me."

"Oh, we've been looking everywhere, and we didn't um . . . um . . . we didn't um . . . recognize you."

"That's okay," I said. "I'll look much better tonight, that is, if I can buy some makeup before I do the show."

I was assured the studio was equipped with a full makeup department. All well and good.

The limousine driver explained the airport mixup.

"The producers told me they were looking for a beautiful blond girl," he said. "And when they saw you they said, 'No, it couldn't be.'"

I collapsed with laughter. "He's quite right," I said. "It couldn't be. However, I am still blond. You wait and see. Tonight with my makeup on and if my luggage arrives, I'll give some semblance of beauty. It will only be an illusion perhaps, but I'll give it my best shot."

At the hotel we ordered a delicious dinner and a good bottle of wine. It arrived two minutes before we had to leave for the studio. We left the wine on the table and bolted down our meal and sped away. The driver dropped us at the wrong entrance and I suffered the humiliation of arriving and mixing with the audience with no makeup, dressed in a black track suit and Reeboks. I didn't even have dark glasses to hide behind. I noticed a few curious stares of disbelief from the crowd before running the perimeter of the building to find a stage door.

"Here I am," I said to the stage manager.

"Who are you?" he demanded.

"I'm Jill Ireland. I'm on your show tonight."

He looked dubious. "Do you need the makeup department?"

"I certainly do."

The makeup woman rolled up her sleeves.

"Oh, no. I'd really rather do it myself. I do my own makeup. I don't feel like myself if somebody else does it."

This offended her. I asked for a magnifying mirror. She didn't have one.

"God, I'm so farsighted I'll have to make my face up in braille," I said.

"I've never been asked for one before," she snipped.

I was losing patience. "Then you can never say that again, can you?" I offered. "Frankly, I've never seen a professional makeup person without one. Do you have a makeup sponge?"

Grudgingly she fumbled through her supplies and found a dirty one.

"A clean one?" I asked.

She ran some alcohol through the soiled sponge. "Now it's clean," she said.

Sue expected me to get up and walk out. No. I'd come so far to talk to people who were waiting to see me, people who needed to hear what I had to say. Not going on would have offended me as a professional. I wanted to prove I was still alive and kicking after my cancer, and I had to look my best.

Suddenly through the door came a bag with my black tuxedo and other clothes. Good! Using the dubious sponge I put on a foundation, powder, used some blusher in a strange shade, blended it in and looked for an eyebrow pencil. I found one, aware it is not hygienic to use secondhand eye makeup. In twenty minutes I had my face on, borrowed hair spray to spritz my hair and primp it up. All things considered, I didn't look bad, and after I donned the black tuxedo I actually looked quite dapper.

I did the show, telling the audience how the producers looked for a beautiful blond at the airport and I hadn't fit the bill. They laughed. But what I liked best was the question-and-answer segment with the audience, looking at people and making real contact.

Afterward I was completely exhausted. Charlie was in Vermont on vacation and I was eager to join him. We loaded ourselves into the limousine with our luggage, all of which finally arrived, and drove to Vermont.

I slept most of the way, during which time I incubated a Hong Kong flu germ. We arrived at four-thirty in the morning. I was happy to be back at Zuleika Farm.

My schedule provided for a three-day respite before taking off for Columbus, Ohio. Charlie came out of the garage to help with the luggage, his eyes heavy with sleep. The frosty air bit into me as I left the warm car.

"Hi," I said, giving him a hug. "God, it's great to be here."

I took a deep breath of the cold night air, which was rapidly becoming cold morning air. Then I entered the house, blissfully unaware that the flu was gaining ground. It struck twenty-five hours after my arrival.

My temperature raged; I ached all over. Light hurt. My hair hurt. I vomited for hours, but found time to thank the fates for at least waiting until I reached the farm. I spent three days drifting in and out of an hallucinatory state. Thoughts floated temptingly around my brain, saying, "Catch me if you can. I may not be around for a while. Come along for the ride; what have you got to lose?"

I had bought the ticket so I climbed aboard.

One scene was crystal clear. It was five or six years earlier and I was looking for birthday presents for Zuleika and my niece Lindsay. I was in a Fred Segal's store shopping for small denim jackets, skirts, and colorful shirts. Disco music blared, making conversation impossible.

As I searched through the racks I heard good-natured laughter behind me and turned to see that my father, bored with waiting, had left his chair and was now dancing to the beat and drawing quite a crowd. Two young male shop assistants with long curly hair and dangling earrings danced with Daddy, saying, "Come on, Grandpa, get down."

And Grandpa was getting down, wiggling his hips and snapping the fingers of his one good hand. I took my purchases to the cashier's desk. Daddy cocked his head and looked at me challengingly. "Lo lo lo," he said, and waved his left arm toward me in invitation.

So I joined them, dancing to the music of Diana Ross . . . or was it Michael Jackson?

"He's so cute, he reminds me of my own grandfather," one youth said.

And Daddy did look cute, in a very up-to-date manner for an English gentleman of his years. He wore Fred Segal blue jeans with bright red suspenders and a denim shirt, his Reeboks fastened with Velcro. I knew he was having more fun than watching me shop, but I found the dancing more strenuous than it looked. I tired quickly and sank into the chair Daddy had vacated. I looked up at my father, making contact with his brown eyes.

"Go for it, Daddy," I said.

My shirt was sticking to me, soaked with sweat. My hair was wet. Someone was wiping my face. I looked up at Daddy, who was spoon feeding me ice chips. His face dissolved into Charlie's concerned one.

"Easy, babe, keep the ice in your mouth," Charlie said. "The doctor said only one chip at a time. You don't want to vomit again."

Then he went back to his deep red-velvet chair, putting his feet on the footrest. The chair sat in a corner of the room in deep shadow.

Before I drifted away again, I realized I hadn't been dreaming, but recalling a scene that had indeed taken place. I sank again into hallucination.

Jason as a five-year-old floated into view. I saw him again as a brave, manly little boy in a doctor's office where

I had brought him to have blood drawn. Paul and I sat on either side of him as the doctor took his small arm, inserted the needle, and pulled blood into the syringe. I was close to tears and Paul was horrified.

Jason, although frightened, put up a manly front, only averting his head at the last moment to cover his eyes with his free hand. He cried quietly. He looked like a grieving man, not a little boy at all.

The vision left me and through the mists and fog I saw myself telephoning my mother in Eastbourne.

The phone rang longer than usual I thought. Finally, my mother answered. "Hello, Mummy."

She replied with her usual, "Hello, Jillie, are you well?"

I sensed she was trying to bottom-line it. "Are you busy, Mummy?"

"Oh, yes, we're watching you on *Shane*. You're so ill, you're dying of swamp fever and you need quinine."

"Oh, well, Mummy, this is serious. I better let you go."

"Oh, no, no, wait a minute, here comes your father. He's getting out of his chair and here he is now."

"Lo lo, lo lo, lo lo," a very excited Jack said. I could tell he was enjoying the show.

"Okay, Dad, good-bye."

The telephone was unceremoniously handed back to my mother, who said a hasty good-bye to her daughter so she could hurry back to her TV set to watch me battle swamp fever on a show that was at least fifteen years old.

The picture melted away.

It was one-thirty in the morning and my mind cleared enough to watch the waning full moon shine whitely, reflecting on the Vermont snow, lighting the bedroom in bright contrasts of black and white. Everything was in sharp focus, including my thoughts, heightened with fever into moon madness.

I knew I was on a fourteen-city book tour, talking and traveling to thirteen American states and two Canadian province, but my thoughts dissolved and I closed my eyes and let the fever run its course.

"Good morning," Charlie said, smiling at me. "Your fever's broken."

He put a thermometer in my mouth. My lips were dry and parched, but I felt much better. Charlie withdrew the thermometer.

"Your temperature is down to one hundred. Would you like to brush your teeth and wash up? It's warm in the bathroom. I'm going to change the sheets."

I looked at Charlie wistfully.

"Do you think it would be all right if I took a quick bath? It would make me feel so much better."

"Okay, baby, but don't linger, and don't get your head wet. After I make the bed, I'll fix you a cup of tea."

"Oh, lovely. Thank you."

I sank into a warm bath and soaked, washing away the illness of the past three days. I took a sweet-smelling nightgown from a large chest of drawers perfumed with sachets. Then I climbed into the clean sheets. Charlie was being most kind. My head pounded from exertion and I was weak. But I sank into my pillows and enjoyed the feeling of fresh well-being.

47
Kier Calls

Jason was like twelve men fighting in a paper bag.

He wanted to straighten out his life. He wanted to work. But his conflict with Kier remained to be solved.

Whenever Jason was offered a job, Kier panicked. He could never let it happen. He sent out louder baby distress signals. Kier was frightened to succeed. If he did, then she would not need to pick him up. She would not come. Kier could not stand up and walk alone. He did not dare be independent, complete, a man. In the doing, he would lose the only link he had, the only signal he knew how to make for her attention—his infant cries, "Mother! Mother! Mother! Hold me. Hold me. I need you."

Like a fish in the ocean Kier sent out distress signals while Jason thrashed helplessly. But no one came.

48
Strays

The book tour was behind me and it was time to face reality and responsibility again.

I headed straight for the beach house. It was eight o'clock in the evening and I was sitting on the porch, looking at a full October moon shining on the inky black breakers as they crashed onto the sand. Somewhere in England it was six o'clock in the morning. In a nursing home where he didn't belong, my father lay in his bed asleep. I pictured him in my mind, his white head on a pillow, his glasses on the bedside table along with his hearing aid. I hoped he dreamed of his youth.

In a small house this same hour, my mother also rested in bed.

"Oh, Mummy, I hope you're feeling better."

I spoke the words aloud, "Sleep well, Mummy; sleep well, Daddy, under your separate roofs."

Somewhere in the California evening a black-haired, blue-eyed, six-foot young man roamed the city restlessly, strung out and hung over, a lonely, haunted figure with only five dollars to his name, and that only if he hadn't bought cigarettes. He is my son, my love, my pain. Jason. I suffer because I have an alcohol- and drug-addicted son and much loved elderly parents in a far-off land, out of reach of my touch. As out of reach as my son, the night prowler. I am in a vise; I cannot extricate myself. I can see no solution.

I had expected to be served a subpoena upon my arrival in Los Angeles. I would be asked to testify in the child custody case involving Lesley-Anne Down, the actress, and her director husband, William Friedkin. It was an ugly battle with both spending a great deal of money trying to prove the other was an unfit parent. I, being so much a parent, was asked to provide fuel for a fire that burned dangerously close to one of my children, Jason.

Jason was being sought by Friedkin, who wanted to seize his son by using mine. Jason had been hiding for six months, living nervously, avoiding being called to testify that as a youngster he had smoked marijuana with Lesley-Anne when the Friedkins were our next-door neighbors. Jason called Friedkin "Billy" and played basketball with him. When Billy asked to see Jason six months earlier he had gone off willingly in hopes Friedkin might offer him a job. Instead, the director asked him to testify that Lesley-Anne was an unfit mother to their small son Jack.

Jason would have to present himself in court as a user of illegal substances. Although my son is a drug addict, at the time Friedkin called he was a recovering addict of about two months. Emaciated and with constant leg cramps, Jason had been fighting hard to stay sober. It was apparent to me that in trying to save his own son from what he thought was unsuitable decadence, Friedkin was pushing my son to the brink.

I had arrived at home to bad news. Charlie had been protecting me from Jason's recent misadventures, jail, and fifteen-hundred-dollars bail for disorderly conduct in a fight with waiters at a Sunset Strip restaurant that catered to the entertainment business. And there was a warrant out for my arrest, hit and run.

Hera, a friend of Jason's, had borrowed my Jeep, which Jason was using, and hit a parked car, which in turn smashed into two other parked cars. Two whiplash suits were pending. Hera had taken off before the police arrived and was now presumed hiding out with Jason. The car, of course, was registered in my name.

One night shortly after my return I received a call from Moira, Jason's ex-girlfriend. In her young child's voice she told me she had seen Jason. "He is living with his friends," she said. "They're just poor, sick drug addicts. But they do try to take care of each other. I've never seen Jason worse. He's thin and sick."

I lay in bed trying to keep calm. The telephone rang. It was Jason. He said I had not heard from him because he was in jail. He apologized and said he was flying to New York on the red-eye that night.

I heard the shake in his voice, the effort to be cocky, belligerent, but he could not quite pull it off.

"Don't go," I said. "Jason, stay here. Come home and eat, please."

"No, Mom, I want to go to New York."

"Jason, stop running. Can't you see you only take your problems with you? I just came back from the East; it's freezing there. And it's just another fucking city."

Jason sounded cold. "Don't swear, Mom. I don't like to hear you swear any more than you like to hear me."

I heard him inhale deeply from a cigarette. I was losing him. He wasn't listening. He was preparing to hang up.

"Jason, you need to go into a hospital."

"No."

"Come home, please."

"Why?" He sounded strung out and exhausted.

"I want you to sleep in a clean bed, have some food, build yourself up."

"I don't want to come home. I can't have visitors after eleven o'clock."

"Jason, bring the girl. It's okay."

"No. I'm going to New York. I'm sick of being arrested."

"Jason, please go to a hospital. Take the girl with you. I'll pay to have you both detoxed. Please."

I heard his mind click. "What?"

"Take the girl. Share a room in the hospital. I will pay for her too."

There was a pause. I heard him inhale his cigarette again. "I'll talk to her."

"Jason, please."

"Okay, Mom. I won't go to New York until tomorrow because of what you said, okay?"

"Come home now, please."

"No. You don't need me coming in at four in the morning. That won't do you any good. I'll call you later."

"Jason, I love you."

"I love you, too, Mom. I'll talk to you tomorrow."

Click. Purr, purr.

I didn't know where he was, and I was getting accustomed to it. I awoke the next morning cold in my bed. I took a pillow and wedged it against my back, wondering why I had such a dull ache in the pit of my stomach. Then I remembered the nightmare I was part of. Jason.

I got up from my comfortable bed and wondered where Jason had slept last night. I soon found out.

Downstairs I fixed myself a cup of tea, sniffing at the front door. No telltale scent of Cartier and cigarettes. No scent outside his room. No scent meant no Jason. I tried his door. It was locked. I entered the small, unlocked adjoining room and walked through the connecting bathroom. Still no scent. I pushed open the door to his room and there was my son. The heat was on and the room stifling. Next to him lay a small, brown-haired girl.

They were both naked, as if they had come in and merely

taken off their clothes in exhaustion before crawling into the big, clean bed. They were emaciated, hip bones jutting sharply. Jason was sleeping as he had all his life, his head arched back to make breathing easier, his dark hair a sharp contrast on the white pillow.

The girl's face was hidden, but I could see she was small, young, and exceedingly thin. I knew they would sleep all day. But he was home. I had my hands on him again. God, how I wished I could brick up the exits to that room.

I had told him I would pay to detox the girl, the same girl who had used my car to hit and run, leaving me holding the bag. But I couldn't find it in my heart to be angry with this small, wounded child. I cursed the drugs that had brought us all to this point, and once again I cursed Janet Berkoff, the woman who had introduced Jason to cocaine at the age of fifteen.

I left Jason and the naked girl in bed, knowing they would not get up until four o'clock or later in the afternoon, a common pattern with drug addicts. I telephoned a friend, Stanley Baker, a recovering alcoholic and an ex-drug abuser. He agreed to come to the Bell Air house after dinner to help.

Two hours before dinner I found Hera in Jason's room. She was dressed in a man's black V-necked cashmere sweater over a boy's shirt. She was desperately thin and had turned up the collar around her face to make herself look less ill. Hera was brushing her hair to appear more presentable. She had impeccable manners and the deportment of a lady. She also appeared to be highly intelligent and well-educated. Dinner was conducted in an orderly fashion with the entire family present. Zuleika and Katrina kept the conversation politely moving, trying not to stare at the two emaciated, drug-addicted people sitting with them at table. Everyone was warm and pleasant toward them. Hera's good manners seemed to get her through the dinner.

Afterward I asked Hera, "Would you like to have a talk?"

I took her into the sitting room and the two of us sat

down for a time. Jason made nervous appearances at the door now and then to see what was going on, trying to lure Hera back into his room. But Hera wanted to talk.

"I would like to explain what happened," she said. "I feel just terrible about the automobile wreck."

"I don't want to hear about that right now, Hera. I'm more concerned about you and Jason and whether or not I can get you to go into a hospital to detox."

During the next hour I used every last drop of my energy to persuade the young woman, who looked to me to be about twenty-eight, to go to a hospital. I told her I would pay her way.

Stanley Baker arrived. "Where's Jason?" he asked.

"In his room," I said. "Let's get him."

Hera went to Jason's room and returned with my son in twenty minutes, during which time I briefed Stanley on the situation.

"I think I can convince the girl," I told him, "but Jason's a harder nut to crack."

"Well, Jill, we'll see what we can do. Where's Charlie?"

"He's in the study. We'll get his support later."

Jason sat on a couch and stared moodily down at the glass-topped coffee table. Hera sat beside him smoking nervously.

"Well, Jason, you rascal, haven't you had enough yet?"

Stanley went on to say how he tricked his wife with urine specimens. She was sure he was doing drugs and brought him vials in which to urinate so she could have them tested. She handed him the vials at odd times, spot-checking. Stanley was able to go days without drugs and while he was clean he would urinate in many, many vials and keep them in a refrigerator in the basement, one that his wife had forgotten about. Then he planted the vials behind toilet tanks in the bathrooms, so when his wife asked him for a urine specimen, he would give her one of the old vials. With a twinkle in his eye, Stanley said, "It drove that poor woman crazy. She knew I was doing something but she couldn't prove it."

Jason sank farther into malevolent gloom while Hera cheered up somewhat at the prospect of entering the hospital. Finally a bargain was struck. They agreed to be taken to the hospital the following morning by Charlie, who would also pay the bill in advance. Stanley and I, thoroughly exhausted, bid each other good-night, believing we had put Jason on the road to sobriety.

The next morning I watched Hera, terrified yet somehow maintaining her tremulous, fragile dignity, shakily applying her makeup in Jason's bathroom, putting bright spots of pink rouge on her cheeks and combing her skimpy hair. I gave her two of my crystals, saying she should give one to Jason, and then I hugged her.

"I'm frightened," she said.

"I know you are."

I could see a decent human being inside the shell-shocked drug victim. Somebody's daughter, somebody's little baby who had been cradled tenderly. That somebody, I knew, had been dead for two years and the little girl, still remembering her mother's upbringing, was now a drug-addicted victim.

But I told myself perhaps this would be the turning point for Hera and Jason. They would begin the long road back to a decent life at the detox center.

Reality was brought home the next evening when I learned that Jason had been kicked out of the hospital after only ten hours. It seemed Jason slipped out of the hospital, found some marijuana, and was discovered by an attendant in bed with Hera smoking pot in the detoxification section.

He and Hera split, and it would be many weeks before I heard from either of them again.

When I did get word, it came in a letter from one of his friends. The writer said he didn't want to interfere, but he knew that Jason was in terrible straits, desperately ill with a flare-up of hepatitis. He was living in a dreadful sort of flop house, the Crescent Hotel, less than a block from the Beverly Hills Police Station. Jason's friend provided the telephone number.

I gave Jason three or four days to bottom out. I grew alarmed when his friend called to say Jason had left the hotel and no one, including Hera, knew where he had gone. I later learned he had slept on a park bench and it was Jason himself who told me that was the night he genuinely hit bottom. He was paranoid, waiting for the police to break in, and he was thoroughly disgusted with Hera, who continually freebased and cried for her dead mother.

Moria telephoned to say she had seen Jason at the hotel. I was beginning to fathom the strange subculture that almost always knew where to find my son—Moira, her younger brother, Charlie John, and Manfred, who had written the letter.

I confided in Valentine a couple of days later that I knew Jason's whereabouts. He and Paul took their brother some food at the Crescent Hotel and returned with dismal stories.

"He looks terrible, Mom."

"His eyeballs are yellow."

"He's in pain and he's sick and really skinny."

"We've got to do something."

I steeled myself. "I'm going to wait."

I had asked the boys not to tell their brother or Charlie that I knew where he was, and they hadn't. Jason assumed all I knew was that he was still just out there. I waited a further week, then could bear it no longer. I telephoned the hotel and a foreign-sounding voice answered.

"May I speak to Jason?" I asked.

He put me right through.

"Hello, Jason?"

"Yeah . . . hello," a voice said.

"This is your mother. Why don't you throw all your things in a pillowcase and meet me?"

Jason said, "I don't have any things. And I don't have any money."

"I'll meet you outside the hotel."

Jason said Hera was doing heavy drugs constantly.

"I can't do anything for Hera now, Jason. I just want to do something for you, please."

"I've been straight for five days, Mom. I've been completely straight. I don't have money for drugs. I don't have money to pay the hotel bill."

"Just meet me out front."

"How long?"

"Fifteen minutes," I said.

"Just give me time to shower, Mom."

"Fifteen minutes," I said.

I drove to the seedy hotel, a hangout for junkies and alcoholics and those who were just plain down on their luck.

My son, because he was so thin, looked even taller than his six feet. He was dressed in clothes I had never seen before and hoped I'd never see again. They were so dirty and ill-fitting I could hardly tell the color.

Strangely and yet typically enough, he was wearing bright white, brand-new sneakers.

"Where did you get the shoes, Jason?"

"I bought them last week."

I thought, How strange. He's starving, he's ill, he has no money for anything, yet somehow he found the money to buy himself new sneakers. Jason had always liked sneakers.

I drove Jason around the corner to a store where I bought him clean khaki slacks and a dark-green cotton shirt.

"Would you like something to eat?" I asked.

"I certainly would," he said.

"Let's stop at The Ginger Man. Let's show the people there that you're clean."

I bought Jason a big meal. The girl behind the bar recognized my son and over the top of his head she mouthed, "Is he in detox?"

"Going to be," I mouthed back.

When Jason went to buy cigarettes, I asked the girl, "Do you know him well?"

"Oh, yes. It's such a tragedy. He sits on this barstool night after night. I'm so glad you're going to do something about it. He's a good person."

Once we were back in the car I used the automobile phone to call Ray Weston.

"Ray, I've got Jason in the car and I want to hospitalize him. I don't want you to tell Charlie."

"Jesus Christ," said Ray. "How am I going to do that?"

"I don't know, but Charlie doesn't need the stress right now, and Jason doesn't need the pressure. I want to hospitalize him for his hepatitis."

"Where are you?"

"On the way to Cedars. Can you call ahead for me?"

Ray did, and Jason was duly registered into a small room where doctors would deal with his chronic hepatitis. He did not need detoxing; he had done that for himself.

Within a week Jason put on weight and to all extents appeared more like a normal, healthy twenty-four-year-old male, except for chronic pains in his legs. That frightened me because they reminded me of the pains Alan Marshall suffered from the medication given him to fight the AIDS virus. Jason was given a battery of tests to establish he had not contracted AIDS from hypodermic needles. His liver was in bad shape, but Ray assured me it would heal as the poisons left his body.

By the time Jason was ready to leave Cedars, I told Charlie what had happened and he graciously allowed him to come home. And so we started another period in Jason's ongoing pursuit of sobriety.

49
Frozen

Kier is like a street accident, sitting stunned in the road, having been hit by a truck. Hit and run. No one saw and he did not know what occurred. He sat, shocked. What happened?

People, seeing him frozen, begin to shout.

"What are you doing?"

"Look, he's sitting in the street!"

"Get out of our way!"

No one could see he was hurt. No one saw the impact. Now the street is clear and innocent looking.

Some try to help him to his feet. But he's too disoriented. He falls down again.

Others shout abuse.

"Bum!"

"Drunk!"

"Bad person!"

Kier is angry but he does not know what hit him. He senses his anger is not justified. He feels guilty. He's being delivered an injustice. But what?"

He is sitting on a pretty street, civilized. Everybody is doing well. Everybody but him, and he can't get up.

He's frozen.

Can't understand why he feels the way he does, why he experiences such dark, black fear.

No one understands. All he hears are lectures, examples, you-shoulds. And he tries. He leans on willing souls, rising only to fall again, each time more bemused, more hopeless, alone, isolated, craving.

He cries, blows bubbles from his lips. Tears flow unheeded down his cheeks. He calls in a language misunderstood: "Mother. Mother."

She doesn't hear. She doesn't know. His new mother hears. She sees. She tries with all her strength to raise him up. She attempts to get the attention of passersby.

"This man's hurt. Help me. Help him."

But they sneer.

"He's drunk."

"He's a drug addict."

"Give up before he drags you down."

She can't. She won't. She sees his innocence, knows him like pieces from a jigsaw puzzle, knows each piece.

With two claps of her hands she could put him together. She can see each fragmented bit and sometimes she does put him together, bracing the picture with her hands to keep it all of a piece, a whole. But when she carefully eases her hands away, the picture shatters. Pieces fly apart. He's back down again.

She thinks, If only. If only she can find a means to glue the bits together permanently.

She asks him if he would like to see his real mother. He thinks about it.

"Maybe she will hold you," she tells him. "Maybe that will make it right. The chemistry, the smell, the feel."

He thinks a long time, longingly, then says, "No, leave her alone. Let her think that at least one of us is all right."

His new mother weeps. Seeing him, she loves him. She

hurts. Oh, how it hurts to watch his efforts, to know his innocence, to feel her culpability. She mourns his life. Never will she give up. Never.

He looks at her with confused, suffering eyes, mute. He doesn't know. He doesn't know it is all right for him to rage. It's just that they hurt him. But he can't know. He can only sit frozen, like a man in the stock. He rages, cries, and feels guilty, and he tries.

But he's frozen.

50
Check and Mate

1987

The contrast in parenting was never more apparent to me than in a nonconfrontational conversation between Charlie and me attempting to come to terms with Jason's chronic pattern of drug episodes interspersed with periods of sobriety.

From the moment our discussion began Charlie assumed the male stance, a firm conviction that boys did not become men by what he considered mollycoddling, although he did keep an open mind. I, on the other hand, immediately assumed the traditional female role of nurturer. The dominant male and his sink-or-swim philosophy, diametrically opposed to female protectiveness, sheltering her wounded offspring to the end.

Charlie was seated comfortably in his chair in our bedroom. I was sitting on the bed with my back against the headboard trying to read, but my mind would not let go and allow me to lose myself in fiction when ever-present facts were so alive, dancing in my brain. I had to share.

I spoke to Charlie, who, a little exasperated with being

interrupted, put his finger on his place in the book and looked up at me.

"Charlie," I said, "I'm thinking about Jason. It's frustrating watching him wriggling and struggling with himself. Every time I try to help him he says, 'No. I've got to find it myself. I know I haven't got anything going for me. I know I have dyslexia and that I can't read and write properly.' He gets so depressed."

Charlie, realizing there would be no more reading for awhile, put his book aside and looked at me levelly. "When you do it alone, you take a longer road."

I said, "I told Jason not one man or woman on earth makes it alone. Everyone has a teacher, a friend, or a guru. I asked if he thought he was so unique he could be the only person in the world to work problems out by himself."

Charlie, heaving a sigh, said, "Point out to him that so far he hasn't worked it out. Tell him he has to have help."

"I have. I told him he had made a complete mess of it doing things his way. The last time we talked he said, 'I know I have. But I'm straight, Mom. I'm sober. I've gone through a lot this week but I haven't done any drugs. Things have come along and I haven't been proud of myself, but I'm still sober.'"

The straws were there to be grasped and Jason and I were grabbing.

"He was frightened, Charlie. He told me that I didn't know what it was like to be out there without drugs. Then I said I do know what it's like. I don't take drugs.

"Charlie, do you know what he told me? Do you remember how he begged us to let him go to the Rolling Stones concert with Chris Jones? Remember her? The tutor? Well, Jason said he was lucky enough to have Chris take him backstage after the concert because one of her friends had something to do with the show. I don't know what it was. While they waited to see the Stones one of their bodyguards gave Jason cocaine. Can you imagine, Charlie! Jason was only ten years old. He absolutely hero-worshiped the Stones.

"Do you remember that T-shirt he got that night, the bright-red one with the big tongue sticking out on the front of it?"

Charlie muttered, "I remember."

I continued, "Jason told me that Keith Richards discovered what had happened and fired the bodyguard."

Charlie looked at me coolly. "You don't know if all that's true."

"I know it is. Jason wouldn't say so otherwise. When I think of how much love and care I put into Jason and that other people took my trust and love and twisted it and left me with the results, I get furious."

I began to feel a knot of tension between my brows. I knew I was frowning and I worked the first two fingers of my left hand in a circular motion, trying to smooth out the furrow.

I was determined not to cry. I wanted to have at least one salt-free conversation with Charlie on this subject.

"He sought it, too, Jill," Charlie said. "He always did what he wanted to do."

Once more taking up the role of placater, I explained for Jason, "He may have sought it, but all children seek fun and pleasure. Older people are supposed to help them. It's an obligation for adults to guide children away from dangers like drugs."

"I think it was another kid that started him."

I said, "I'm sure it was an older kid."

"Probably one of his peers," Charlie said.

The familiar two-step had started between us.

"You know, Charlie, Jason never went through adolescence. He never grew up. He understands this. He told me he knows he has to grow up now."

"He's told me similar stories. He needs help, but he refuses to go back to the psychiatrist."

"Jason's just angry because of some of the things Dr.

Brovar said when I was there." Dr. Brovar was a psychiatrist, specializing in drug addicts and alcoholics, whom Jason had been seeing.

"That's only an excuse."

"He says he's trying to sort his mind out after what happened the one day I visited Brovar with him."

"He's using that day to break an appointment. He doesn't want to go back."

"I told him we had a deal. If I paid for the hospital and he got well, then he would go to Brovar faithfully."

"If he stops going to Brovar, he will stop everything else, one at a time, until he's back on drugs," said Charlie.

"How can I *make* him go back to Brovar?"

"You tell him we had a deal, then threaten him. Say 'Out, Jason. I don't want to be responsible for you in any way, shape, or form. If I hold up my end of the deal, you must hold up yours.'"

"He's so angry at Brovar, he wouldn't agree."

"Jason can't face being told who he really is."

"I know that and he knows it too. Should I tell him you will kick him out if he doesn't go back to the doctor?" I asked.

"Tell him that."

"Then he will stay with his friend Johnny for a few days, and then another of his friends."

"That's all right."

"But during that time he might just start . . . right now he's trying to handle his frustration on his own, in his room at home."

"He's looking for an excuse to do what he wants to do. Now if it's drugs he wants, he's waiting for us to make this move, for me to kick him out."

I began to flounder; treading water was becoming increasingly fatiguing by the minute. I lifted my chin higher. "Then I don't want to make that move."

"Give up. But it won't make any difference, because if

he's looking for a reason, he'll find it whether you are part of it or not."

A straw floated by. I reached for it. "I find if I go slowly with him, I make headway, as I did in my conversation with him last night."

"I don't go by those conversations. They don't mean anything to him. Jason is a real con artist. He's not very good at it, but he's been operating on the con for a long, long time."

Now I was getting desperate, defensive. I was caught up in a current I couldn't overcome. I tried anyway. "But he also cares. He wants respect, a job, family . . ."

Charlie shot back, "Don't you see how dumb that sounds? Everybody wants respect. I want this, I want that."

"But he's not *had* respect. Nobody respects him. He knows that."

"I know; I told him."

"I'm aware of that."

"Yeah. It's just like talking to you right now. It passes time. Now another day has gone by. He's going to go on this way."

Charlie picked up his book and I went back to the knot in my brow. But, typically, I had more to say.

"Jason wants to work for a music-recording studio in Florida. He impressed the owners. He loves music, but he doesn't know the first thing about it. Jason's very imaginative and is great talking sometimes. I offered to send him to school to learn about sound techniques."

Charlie glanced up. "It wouldn't help. He can't possibly study."

"Why?"

Charlie put down his book for a second time. "Because it's so complicated. You have to learn to handle sophisticated electronic gear. He just couldn't do it. He thinks it is just pushing switches while listening to music through earphones."

"So we have to tell him again that he can't do it. But I wish there were something, some way, Charlie."

I paused a moment, then said, "We can't just throw him away."

"He's throwing himself away."

"Yes, but that's because he wants to be someone else. He doesn't want to be this person. He desperately wants to become a man."

Charlie replied, "If he wanted respect and to be a man and stand on his own two feet, he would straighten up. Right now, all he's looking for is sympathy from you. He wants pity and sympathy, and that's it."

"It's terrible. I can't help loving him, though, Charlie."

"It's difficult for me because I'm trying to find something about him to love. He makes me laugh now and again, but then he takes it away. You see, I'm a male and he's male, so it makes a difference."

"You have a lot more patience with the opposite sex. So do I. It's the way it is. But you can identify with the same sex, like I identify with Katrina."

"Yes, I can identify with him," Charlie said. "I remember him as a kid, and he was always different from the others. He was the one that disobeyed all the time."

"It said in that book you read about drug addiction that disobeying the rules is a trait of the addictive personality."

Charlie said, "Yes. Jason's hyper. When the family is having fun, Jason needs extra fun. Everything with him is *extra*. A little bit more. He gets excited by taking chances, doing what he shouldn't do. He likes risk, being out of control."

"At least he's come to grips with his dyslexia. He doesn't hide it. That's a big step. He's having to say he's not as good as everyone else. I'm grateful for every little thing he's trying to do. And he's not well. He has a lot of pain."

"I'm not even sure that's true. He might just want to have the drugs, Jill."

"The only drug the doctors are giving him is Somar for his leg cramps."

"He should exercise to build himself up."

With that, I climbed off the bed and went to brush my teeth. Thankfully, Charlie went back to his book.

I returned and got into bed, picked up my book but found myself reading the first four lines over and over again. So I took off my glasses, placed them on the bedside table, and stared at Charlie.

"You said you thought you just raised a boy and that was it, but now we have to raise him all over again. It seems that's true."

Charlie yawned and put his book away. "He's going to fight it the same as he did as a kid."

"There's good in Jason, Charlie."

"Of course there is. A lot of good, but to what extent?"

"Sometimes I give up hope. Other times I hope again that it will be all right. Now, I don't see how it possibly can be. He tells me he wants to be straight with such fervor, but he won't let me help. He's so damn stubborn, but maybe that will help pull him through."

"He doesn't want me to help him get a job because he doesn't want what he says he wants. He doesn't want a job, yet he knows having a job and earning his own way is the way to get respect."

I said: "He doesn't think he could handle the stress of a job right now."

"He's interested in clothes, so let him be a clothing salesman."

"Where?"

Charlie said, "There are signs all over Beverly Hills and Westwood begging for salesmen."

"Maybe they want experience."

"If they can't get experience, they'll take anybody they can get."

"How can you make him go to work? Make him want to try?"

"As long as we treat him the way we're treating him now, he gets along fine."

I asked Charlie what the alternatives were.

"The alternative is you shouldn't have picked him up at the hotel in the first place. He should have ended up in jail or wherever else he was."

"You couldn't let him go to jail. There was a bench warrant out for his arrest and that girl who banged up my Jeep. You couldn't let that go on. Jason would have reached bottom and never come up."

Enigmatically, Charlie said, "Yes, he would."

"But you wouldn't let him go to jail . . ."

"Because the crime wasn't that great."

"What's to keep him from going to jail in the future for breaking probation? I don't think jail is a good idea. I don't think that that would help him because the episode would end up in the *National Enquirer* as just another movie-star's-kid story," I said.

"Jill, it's not that. If Jason went to jail and saw the alternative to what he's doing, it would make a difference. If he hit bottom, being in a tank with a bunch of others for alcoholism or something . . ."

"I was going to let him hit bottom. He was sleeping on park benches."

"He wasn't sleeping on benches."

"He did. Two nights."

"He told you that, didn't he?"

"Okay," I said. "He did."

"Well, then I don't believe him."

"I believe him. Hera said it too, and so did Manfred. I didn't want him in jail because he had chronic hepatitis and he was likely to die. I couldn't let that happen."

"It's difficult to discuss. I called Dr. Brovar to make an appointment for Jason and he said, 'Jason is a scammer.'"

"But he's also said a lot of good things about Jason."

Charlie came to his feet and got in bed beside me. "Are you going to read anymore?" he asked.

"No," I replied. "I think I've memorized these four lines."

"All right, then, I'm going to turn off the light. Give me a kiss good-night."

We kissed gently.

"Good-night, Jill."

"Good-night, Charlie."

We had resolved nothing, but in our hearts we knew we would continue to be Jason's support team, hoping, trying, bailing him out. But I think Charlie and I both understood, deep down, that there would never be any quick solutions, any ready answers to the almost insurmountable obstacles that stood in the way of our son's striving toward manhood and respect.

Only a few months later Charlie told Jason to move out and get himself an apartment, for which my husband would pay considerable rent.

I was so naïve, I loved my son so much, I actually hoped his proposal didn't hurt Jason's feelings. I realized Jason's pain was mine, even after I had resolved to let go with love, let go of this child of mine who orbited my center like a glowing, shrieking foreign moon.

Everyone told me he had to hit bottom. The thought chilled me. He might hit bottom and never come up again. Then Jason disappeared for three days. He had been emaciated, not an ounce of fat anywhere on his body, his face narrow, gaunt, and his eyes bloodshot and sunken. Blisters festered his gums. The once-tight jeans hung on his sticklike legs. His buttocks were flat, almost nonexistent.

I imagined him in situations with drug users, his energy burning as if through a plain of dry grass, destroying his life's potential, his health, his soul. Then, as I sank into submissive abjection, Jason turned up. I saw the beat-up old

Bronco in the driveway, blocking the path of two automobiles. My heart leaped with happiness. He'd made it home. Jason was home.

I bid a hasty hello to Charlie through the study door and walked quickly through the corridor to the boys' wing, passing photographs of the family, pictures taken in France, London, Istanbul. The aroma of Cartier perfume and cigarette smoke told me Jason was in his room. He was lying quietly on his bed. I put my hand on his cheek. It felt somewhat fuller, covered with a thick, black stubble. His eyes were bloodshot.

"Are you napping, darling?"

"No, Mom."

"Jason, I would like to talk to you, now, while you're peaceful."

I sat on the bed, resting my back against the wall. "Did you find my note?"

"Yes," he replied noncommittally.

I had written a letter trying to put into words my feelings about sobriety.

A copy of *Life Wish* was on the bedstand. "Will you read my book?"

"Yes, I'm going to." Then his face brightened with sincere pleasure. "It's in a store in Westwood already. I saw it on display."

The happiness vanished as quickly as it appeared as I watched, my emotions quietly on hold.

"What are you going to do about your life?" I asked.

His large blue eyes were childlike, innocent.

"It can't go on," I continued. "I know you are addicted again. I also know you use drugs to mask your pain." I paused, then made up my mind to say something that needed saying. "Darling, I accept you. I know your pain, and I know how hard it is for you to give it all up.

"You've had a dialogue going with drugs for so many years, but it's no good. It's got to stop. It is always the same with you. When you were in first grade it was dyslexia. I can still hear you at five saying, 'I don't want to learn to write; I don't see the point of it.' But you did learn to read and write and you're glad about it now, aren't you?"

His face was soft and young, my bold Jason.

"I know it's fine for a nonaddict to say give it up," I continued. "I know, I can't give up chocolate; I can only imagine the dreadful pull of cocaine, alcohol, and heroin. I want so much to help you. I love you."

He moved off the bed and put his head in my lap and began to cry quietly. I held him until he stopped.

Then, with an abrupt change of mood, he declared himself hungry. We sent out for food. He was quiet and calm. I felt I had reached my son. The wild energy wasn't with him. When the food arrived we shared it, sitting on his bed, happy, close. I felt I had achieved something, satisfied for now to be with him, not lecturing, not pleading.

He pushed spaghetti from the cardboard container onto a plate for me. Then he ate pasta from the box. We shared a chicken sandwich. Jason ate voraciously, no sign of mouth blisters.

"Slowly, Jason, slowly," I said.

I wanted the food to stay down and nourish him. I didn't give a thought to anything but this moment we shared. That was all I had. Oh, how I loved that recalcitrant son of mine. I knew I would never let go, not yet anyway. We had a long way to go before we hit bottom.

51

Veranda

1987

It was always a crushing blow to know that Jason was off the wagon, first with alcohol, then massive doses of cocaine. I remember 1987, before I left for my book tour, when I was on the beach-house veranda gazing at the ocean, thinking how lucky I was. The family was together. Jason had come to have dinner with us. The occasion was Valentine's birthday. After dinner Jason joined me on the veranda, looking out into the night. He said his doctor told him he had only a few months to live.

I can still feel my stomach taking a dive. I was sure he must have AIDS from infected needles used to administer drugs.

"What do you mean, Jason?"

"Well, Mom, the doctor said that I have only a few months left to live if I don't start straightening up. I've screwed up my body so much with all the drugs."

"Don't tell me you're taking drugs again!"

"No, Mom, nothing like that," he said, lying through his teeth.

I gullibly believed him.

"I've got a hole right through my nose, you know, from all the cocaine. My septum's completely ruptured. Here, feel."

He took my hand and tried to force me to waggle his nose. I recoiled. "No, Jason, I don't want to feel."

"And I've been vomiting. I've thrown up blood."

I stared at him. "Jason, if you go back on drugs, I'll do something dreadful. I will do something so terrible to you, you'll never forget it."

He laughed. "Well, Mama, you're some tough lady. Why weren't you like this before?"

"I'm telling you, Jason, I swear to you I will do something terrible if I catch you on drugs again."

I didn't catch him. Months went by. Jason, as usual, avoided me while he was using.

52
Eastbourne

1987

The British publishers of *Life Wish* asked me to fly to London to publicize the book in a series of television, newspaper, and magazine interviews, and I happily accepted. It would mean another opportunity to spend time with my parents.

It would be my first visit to England in two years. Then I had accompanied Charlie as his wife. I was excited and grateful to be alive, but the threat of cancer recurrence was still a very realistic shadow.

This time I was on my own with trusty Sue Overholt helping pave the way. I would spend a week at Eastbourne in the south of England near the sea before doing my party numbers for the media in London.

Jill Ireland was coming home to give her book to my family of Britishers, coming home full of love for my fellow countrymen, hoping to be able to shine a light toward the end of the tunnel as I had been told I had done in my adopted country. I would be bringing something of myself to leave behind, a most personal part of myself, my book.

Even as I thought sentimentally of England and my loved ones there, I had a touch of America pinned to the lapel of my suit. It was Valentine's birthday gift to me, a red, white, and blue glittering rhinestone pin with the three letters *U.S.A.* I could not forget where my life was now.

New York to London on the Concorde, a supersonic three hours and forty minutes! I remembered the old fourteen-hour flights from Los Angeles. I counted my blessings. I loved my life. I would not change anything about it. I wished Jason and Daddy could walk in my shoes for an hour. Especially Jason, so he could see the beauty in the world as I saw it, and Daddy, as a reward for his suffering.

I looked out of the Concorde's window and saw the Rolls-Royce engines controlling our destiny as we flew faster than sound. We built it, we Brits. We make them tough, my mother was fond of saying. Generations of Ireland people, England, Angel Land, Land of the Angels. I'm coming home.

Forgotten was the recent evening with Charlie and Susie Dotan when we watched *Gandhi* on the video machine. I felt a bit like a German watching a film about the Holocaust. Now all I felt was a sentimental, empire loyalist's pride. I felt my British accent thicken, dropping off years of America's burr I'd acquired. Jilly Flower was amongst her own. I was coming home bearing gifts of whiskey, silk, perfume, eye makeup, and a book with my picture on the cover. *Life Wish*, love wish. The girl from Hounslow had stood the test of time and trouble and, as the mirror in the lavatory told me, I was looking good.

As I collected my luggage at Heathrow Airport, I encountered Joan Collins, perfectly made up and looking immaculately elegant in a white-cotton suit and white high-heeled pumps, her legs slender. I felt like a bit of a country bumpkin in my long navy skirt and blazer, tennis shoes and white socks, my face shiny without makeup. I was glad I wore my dark glasses.

"Hello, Joan."

"Hello," she said. "How are you? I just came in on the red-eye and caught the connection with the Concorde."

"God, Joan, I stayed over in New York. I'm too elderly for that. The red-eye! How do you do it? You look band box."

She smiled at me. "I'm older than you."

I liked her. She collected her bags and we said good-bye.

Reg, our driver in London in 1985, met us. He wore the bright-red tie I had given him that Christmas.

On the long ride to Eastbourne I thought about Daddy all the way. It had been thirteen months since I had seen him.

The Grand Hotel Eastbourne welcomed me warmly and soon I rode up in the old elevator to my suite. On the way I passed my parents' room, paused, then knocked on door Number 245.

Mummy answered, looking unchanged since I had seen her last year.

"Ah," she said as we hugged.

Daddy sat watching television, the volume turned high. He looked up as I entered. He wore a red tartan flannel robe and looked smaller than last I'd seen him. He did not get up.

I hugged and kissed my father. He didn't cry as he usually did when he saw me after a long separation. He was changed somehow, a subtle but definite difference since his latest stroke. He did not try to speak. But when he managed to get to his feet, he began singing, one arm extended in the pleading, ingratiating gesture of a professional entertainer.

"Poor little dickie birds out on the sea," he sang.

I was perplexed. He usually sang only when it was appropriate in a singsong around a piano. This was different; it was by way of a greeting. Had Daddy given up speaking words no one understood?

Was he singing because he knew at least those words made sense even though they weren't the ones he wanted to say, the ones in his head? I remembered recently he had only sung to me on the telephone. I looked at my father and joined in. We communicated through Poor Little Dickie Bird's "Oh, dear me."

We ordered tea in my suite. The many fine chains that I wore around my neck, with crystals dangling from them, had become tangled. Mummy proceeded to untangle them while Daddy and I had tea.

"You still look handsome, Daddy," I said.

I became aware he was lip-reading; his hearing had gone almost completely. He was now locked in. No speech, no hearing. But he could sing, by God.

As Mother continued to work on my necklaces I yelled at my father, "You don't think I came all this way to see you, do you!"

Daddy's eyes twinkled.

"Not at all. I came because no one in America could untangle my necklaces, so I had to have my mother do it."

My father laughed. He'd heard and understood.

The fierce fire in his eyes was gone. God, had he given up? No, not he. It was late. Eleven-thirty and well past his bedtime. He was probably tired. Daddy rose.

"Are you going to bed?" I asked challengingly. "Oh, no you don't. I just got here."

He sat down again.

"I have a present for you."

I gave him a royal-blue silk tie from Paris and a bottle of cologne. He expressed pleasure. Then I gave him the Johnnie Walker whiskey, and there it was.

"Ah, lo lo," he bellowed, his eyes snapping with the old fire.

Yes, my dad was pleased with his whiskey. The fire was alight again. He gathered up his new possessions with his one strong arm and made for the bedroom through the connecting door to my suite, stopping just long enough to kiss me.

"Good-night, Daddy."

"Good-night, Jack," my mother said. "I'll see you in a moment. I'm going to untangle these chains."

Soon Mummy went to bed. Overcome by fatigue, I got into bed and slept until 4 A.M. Then I awoke as from an afternoon nap. I was starving and thirsty—jet lag. I called the concierge.

"What can we do for you, Miss Ireland?" a kind male English voice inquired.

"Oh, I'd love some tea."

"I'll make you a pot with pleasure," he said.

"Thank you. And I'm so hungry. It's only eight in the evening in Los Angeles. It's my dinnertime. Could I have some toast?"

"Yes, I'll make you some toast."

"Thank you." Suddenly, tea and toast seemed like a special treat. "Could I have some marmalade too?"

"Yes, ma'am. I'll bring it right up."

"Thank you," I said sincerely. Then I telephoned Charlie.

"What are you doing awake?" he asked.

"Oh, you know how it is. I slept like a log for four hours and now I'm wide awake. How's everything at the house?"

"Fine."

"How's Cassie?"

"She's at the beach house."

"Okay. I love you."

"I love you too."

"My tea is at the door. I'll call you tomorrow. Bye, Charlie."

"Bye, Babe."

The tea was brought in by two very English porters. They treated me as if I were one of their family.

They bid me good day and I settled down with my tray. Snuggled in the hotel bathrobe, I wolfed down the toast and gulped the tea. It was delicious as only a middle-of-the-night snack can be.

Then I looked out the window to watch dawn break over the English Channel. I was home. I was Jill Ireland again.

"Hi, England. I'm back," I whispered, pressing my hands against the damp-feeling windowpane.

Then I pulled the curtains firmly aside and stood back from the window, turning to face the light. I touched the right side of my body where my breast used to be, over the scar that was now not much more than a fine white line, and I thought about reconstructive surgery. I had to admit I had become fond of my scar over the last three years. It stood for something, and it reminded me that I had withstood; and although I had two more years before I would be in remission, I knew at this point I was well. I did not need the medical stamp of approval.

I placed my left hand on my flat, prepubescent chest and then placed my right hand on my left breast, feeling the fullness, the roundness. I looked at the nipple and inspected the nearly invisible one-inch scar that Dr. Mitchell Karlan had left when he performed the lumpectomy eighteen months earlier. I cupped my breast in my hand and tried to remember what it was like to hold two breasts. Incredibly, I could not. I had become quite comfortable with the one side of my flat chest.

Still, it would be wonderful to be able to wear a round neckline or perhaps a strapless gown. The elegant V-necked gowns and off-the-shoulder, just-touching-the-breastbone style had satisfied me for three years, but I was beginning to look wistfully at photographs of the new styles with cleavage.

I could no longer simply slip on a cotton shirt and shorts to go down to the pond in Vermont. It was necessary to fetch a bra and insert the silicone prosthesis. It is a small aggravation, to be sure, compared to the gift of life that the amputation gave me.

I do not want to be a cancer victim forever. God knows, I'd like to be able to forget it. But it is difficult to forget when you take off your clothes and look in the mirror. I see the huge knife wound running from my right armpit to the center of my chest. I knew I could live the rest of my life with this scar, but there was an alternative—a surgical implant.

I remembered the women at the Reach to Recovery Group and how they had shown me their two beautiful breasts. I could not help wondering, though, how I would look in the future with an aged woman's body and two pert teenage breasts. I would have the left one worked on as well, but I'd better not make it too youthful looking. I inspected it closely; it didn't look bad. But did I want to mutilate it by splitting the nipple to make a nipple for my right side? No. I was rather proud of my left breast. At least it showed anyone who was interested what my right one once looked like. Well, you can't have everything.

"Good-night, cruel world," I said, using Charlie's expression but not feeling as if the world were cruel at all. I felt like a spoiled, loved child, my Mummy and Daddy in the next room, and my tummy full with a hot drink. I jumped back into bed and went to sleep.

53

Runaway

1987

I awoke at one-thirty in the afternoon and fixed myself a cup of tea, using the electric kettle my mother had brought along. From the balcony I saw my parents sitting under an umbrella beside the swimming pool.

"Daddy," I called. My mother looked up and called my father's attention to me. He rose immediately and I could tell we were off and running.

Soon he was at my door with a beatific smile. Mummy appeared looking terribly English in a cotton skirt and blouse covered by a green cardigan. "Good morning, Jilly. We've had lunch. I had a sandwich and all Dad wanted was a coffee."

I roused Sue from her jet-lagged slumbers. "Come on, Sue, we're going shopping."

We decided to take a taxi to the center of Eastbourne and walk back. Mummy protested: "He walks so slowly he'll never make it back."

But my father was adamant. "Yush," he said with a definite nod of his head.

Daddy was out of the cab and into the store before I could pay the driver. We bought a few items and set out on the two-mile walk to the hotel. Daddy strutted ahead.

"Are you sure you can make it, Daddy?" I asked after fifteen minutes. He looked tired. His eyes were bloodshot and his mouth was open, but he kept going.

"Slow down, Dad; Mummy can't keep up," I pleaded. But a curt shake of his white head declared it was her problem; he was forging on.

The seafront was crowded with people of my parents' generation, sitting or walking their way through their golden years. A few elderly couples were holding hands. Some chatted quietly.

We walked at beach level, some six feet below the deck-chair tier where hundreds of chairs contained mostly elderly, prim Englishwomen. Their dignity was unconsciously shattered in every case from our point of view by an array of stockinged legs and pastel bloomers. In their enjoyment of the sun on their limbs a thousand proper Englishwomen were quite unaware of exposing their thighs and knickers in the boldest of ways. Fortunately, tourists are rare in Eastbourne and Englishmen would not have taken any notice whatsoever.

Feeling mischievous, and out of earshot of my mother, I whispered to Sue, "I believe the name of this stretch of the strand is Crotch Walk."

We giggled and then I called out to my father, "Look, Daddy, there's an empty bench. Let's sit awhile."

No. Nothing doing.

My mother, though, sat down. My father had awakened her at six and then locked himself in the bathroom. Poor Dorothy had had to call a porter to get him out. Now she watched him march away into the crowds. She muttered that she wished she had left him locked up.

"Let him go, Jill. He'll find his way, or else we'll catch up with him when I get my breath."

"That will teach you to say he's slow," I told her.

My father and his blue sports jacket disappeared into the crowd of white heads, just another old man, albeit a stubborn one, walking alone.

Sue, Mummy, and I sat for five minutes and then decided to move on.

There was no sign of Daddy ahead of us nor in any of the empty chairs we passed along the way. I teased Mummy about her weekly visits to Eastbourne.

"Every Wednesday I come here," she said, "and sit down after shopping to listen to the band." She pointed to a bandstand. "Of course it plays only in the summer."

"Do you come here alone, Mummy?"

"Yes, but I sometimes flirt with a nice man if there is one."

"Good for you, Mummy."

I felt sad for my mother. I could see her valiantly sitting alone amongst the couples and singing with the band.

Music could be heard through speakers. A recording played an old Welsh song that I remembered from my girlhood.

There'll always be a welcome in the hillsides,
There'll be a welcome in the dales,
Oh, everywhere there will be singing
When you come home again to Wales.

I felt my eyes fill as I looked at the sparsely filled seats surrounding the bandstand. A few old ladies were already singing along. It was a place where they could all have a singsong.

"Do you sit here by yourself, Mummy?"

"Yes," she said, defying all pity, "and I sing too."

Sue and I proceeded to tell her she needed a Wednesday boyfriend.

"Well, I'm working on it," she replied.

I began picking out prospective candidates for my mother's favors. "There's one, Mummy," I said, pointing out an old gentleman who looked to be in his late seventies. He sat alone on a deck chair looking forlorn and lost. "He looks as if he'd like a girlfriend."

"I don't like the looks of him," my mother said. "I don't like his socks. I'll find one on my own, thank you."

I kept the game going all the way back to the Grand Hotel, my choices becoming more and more outlandish and my mother's reactions more tart.

"How about him?" I questioned, as a once tall, but now bent man of about eighty passed with a terrier on a leash.

"Not bad," replied my mother. "But see, he's already being traipsed down by those two hussies behind him. They've obviously got their eye on him, and they look local to me."

The hussies were two genteel ladies in their seventies with identical white, short fine hair and similar pastel flowered dresses under pale cardigans. One carried a cane. They both wore glasses and were looking sweetly straight ahead.

"Yes, I see what you mean," I said.

Finally, Sue said, "I wonder what happened to Mr. Ireland."

"I expect he found his way to the hotel," I said. But when we arrived, he wasn't there. The concierge hadn't seen him and he was not sitting in the garden, the tea room, or the lounge.

In the bedroom I said, "I bet he went past the hotel."

"No," said Mummy. "He'd see it. How could he miss it?"

I fought the fear that he had had another stroke or heart attack. "Maybe he sat down and fell asleep."

"Maybe," said my mother.

"Well, Mummy, he was determined to walk without us. He had his own way, and that was right. We can't do what he wants all the time; and by the same token, why should he do as we tell him? It's his life; he made his choice."

The minutes ticked by. "Maybe I should call the local hospital. Maybe he fell down. Was he wearing his medal?" I referred to the gold Medic-Alert tag he wore on a chain around his neck with his name and telephone number.

"Oh, yes, he always wears it; but if they phone home, no one's there," she said, stating the obvious. "I wrote the name of this hotel and put it in his pocket. We'd hear if something happened. He'll turn up. He always does."

"Yes, but we'll never know what happened," I said. "He won't be able to tell us."

Then the phone jangled. It was Sue. "The concierge called, Jill. Your father's been picked up by the police. He's at the station. Shall I go get him?"

"No, Sue, I'm not missing this. I'm coming down."

"Neither am I," said Mummy. "I'm coming too."

I could not help but think of the times Jason had been in the police station. Will my two J's, Jack and Jason, ever learn to keep out of trouble? But I kept this thought to myself.

"Second time today Jack's been locked up," said my mother cryptically, remembering the morning bathroom incident.

We took a taxi to the police station and there was my father, locked in a room. When he saw us, he started going *"Ah ah ah . . ."* full throttle.

I couldn't help laughing. "What have they got you in for this time?" I asked. "Drunk and disorderly?"

I asked the police sergeant, who regarded me somewhat askance, "What happened?"

"He was trying to go into the wrong hotel," the sergeant said. "He made a mistake. They didn't know him, so they called us. We didn't find the piece of paper with the Grand Hotel written on it right away."

My mother said, "Well, do we have to sign for him?"

"No," said the sergeant, smiling. "Just take him home."

My father, mustering his dignity, left the police station and climbed into the front seat of the taxi. Sue, my mother, and I were crammed ignominiously together in the back. My mother and I could not stop laughing.

"What are you going to do next, Jack?" she asked. "One more thing and I'm taking a bus home and leaving you with Jill."

"Wait for us next time, Daddy, okay?" I said, patting his shoulder.

"Yush," he replied.

But I knew he wouldn't. He never would. He'd march on ahead for the rest of his life. That was his power.

The publishers had mapped a busy week, averaging five interviews a day, beginning at seven o'clock in the morning. Well, that was why I had come to England. I'd bite the bullet and do my best. I just hoped my health would hold up. Still, with my father for light entertainment, I was assured of a few laughs.

Later, during dinner, I looked at my old man, his serviette tucked beneath his chin, looking so angelic. I was moved to say, "Oh, Daddy, you are so sweet."

He did not understand at first.

"He's not used to being called that," my mother said, amused. "Jack, Jill thinks you're sweet."

"Yes, you are, Daddy. You're so sweet."

He looked pleased and gave my mother a glance as if to say, "There you are, you see, I'm sweet."

His wife smiled tenderly. "No, you're not, Jack. Here, read my lips. You're an old bugger," she said slowly, enunciating. My mother had the last word.

Daddy laughed.

Day one of my English trip was declared over. I awoke once more in the middle of the night, my mind darting about. How much like my father I was, stubborn, willful.

I could see my face in my father's; see myself in his eyes.

I had even lost the hearing in my left ear, as he had. Yes, I was a chip off the old block, all right.

My mother is a strong character too. John and I should have been wimps, I thought. We were reared by Punch and Judy, which John called them because they fought a lot, passionate, steamy fights to which we were witness. The passionate, steamy reconciliations, to which we were not witness, must have been the cement that bonded the relationship I was now watching. Mummy's complete, tender, spunky, and cantankerous devotion to her handicapped, scrofulous old Romeo, Jack Ireland, her handsome, charming, witty husband, allowed him still to rule with an iron fist.

The woman gave him almost as good as she got, and certainly more love than even she comprehended. Yes, she accepted and did for him the very best she could. No matter how hard she struggled in rebellion against his youthful hell-raising and bullying tantrums, the years had made them one. She was his woman, and he knew it; never doubted it.

But I knew my mother had once dreamed of being more than a part of someone else's anatomy. Fate decreed differently. Sometimes I found myself hoping Daddy would die first, leaving her a few years of peace to live just for herself. I hoped in that event she would live with me and Charlie. But I was beginning to see the selfishness of my thoughts.

I was no longer a little girl, and my mother, though she loved me very much, had her own life. My hopes would only make her once more an appendage of a stronger being. She would trade my father and his bullying for mine. Perhaps now, with Daddy afflicted and dependent on her, she was for the first time truly her own woman, having proved she could do everything to run their lives—pay the bills, sign legal documents, take responsibility, make decisions—and while doing it all she kept my father, her husband, a man to be respected, well-dressed, living in his own well-kept home, just as he had earned it by his life's toil.

My mother's one concession was Daddy's once-a-month visit to the nursing home, and that was only so she could keep going.

For many years I urged her to move to California so they would be closer to me.

"I'll get a house for you both, Mummy. Come on," I urged.

Not now. She knew what she was doing, every instinct was surely in place. My mother was mistress of her life now, and she still had her man, her handsome, desirable ladies' man. He was all hers. I couldn't compete with her for my daddy, and I couldn't steer her away from my baby brother. Those days were gone. I had grown up.

I was a witness only to their life's drama, marveling at the strength and personal power that emanated from those two sturdy, quixotic souls surely made for one another. True soul mates. I could see it in their eye contact.

Twice during dinner at the Grand Hotel in Eastbourne that night Daddy had challenged Mummy with his eyes, and I saw her body soften, her eyes acquiesce. All those years of intimacy. They had never gone their separate ways. Never. Never thought of it. They belonged together for as long as God saw fit or until they got it right, whichever came first.

54

"Red Robin" Revisited

The next morning I was awakened at ten by my mother's gentle touch, the first time we had shared such a moment since I was a teenager.

"My mummy's waking me up," I said, stretching. "Good morning."

She told me my father had been up since six-thirty and that she had convinced him to return to bed for another two hours.

"I knew he would just sit and stare for hours," she said. "He can't read a book. He reads the first page over and over again, then forgets what he read. And this morning he broke his electric razor for the third time."

Daddy arrived in a white-and-blue-striped seersucker jacket, a wine shirt, and green tie with wild geese rampant. A snappy dresser, my dad. He watched my breakfast disappear but refused breakfast himself.

Before leaving Los Angeles for Eastbourne a few days earlier, I had spoken to him on the phone. Taking a cue from my mother, who told me that Daddy had gained weight, I said, "Daddy, when I see you, I'm putting you on a diet."

My threat had galvanized him to diet. Since my arrival in England he had refused to eat. I admired his eighty-two-year-old vanity. As the days passed I also enjoyed the new woman-to-woman relationship with my mother. It was pleasant to know her as one woman knows another. I liked her. She was feisty and opinionated, a gutsy, salt-of-the-earth woman.

When I completed my breakfast, Daddy joined Sue and mother in the large airy sitting room of the suite. Through the adjoining doors I heard him sing:

Whistle while you work,
Hitler is a jerk.
So's his army,
They're all balmy,
Whistle while you work.

The song brought memories of my early childhood war years. His next song was of the same vintage:

Hitler has only got one ball,
Goering has one but very small,
Himmler is somewhat sim'lar,
Poor old Goebbels has no balls at all.

God, I was being thrown back to the forties before lunch. Encouraged by Daddy's attempts to communicate through song, I decided to change the mood and test his memory. I sang:

I'm just a kid again,
Doing what I did again,
Singing a song,
When the red, red robin
Comes bob-bob-bobbin' along.

Daddy joined in, bobbing and weaving as he danced to my morning soprano.

"We've changed a bit, old chap, since last we sang that song," I said.

"Yush," said Daddy.

My mother feigned dismay. "Jack, I'm going to have you put down."

"If you do," I said, "have him stuffed and he can sit in my living room."

"All right," Mummy said. "Yes, Jack, you can sit there and watch what everyone is up to."

"Shall I stuff you too, Mother?"

"No. I wouldn't want that. I hope to go while I sleep."

"You're not ready to go yet, are you, Mummy?"

"Well, sometimes I think I am."

I'd heard this from her before. I said, "I'm sorry to tell you, but I'm very intuitive and I'm afraid you'll live to be a hundred."

"Oh, Jill, shut up. I don't want to be a hundred."

"Yes, you do. Once Daddy's put down and stuffed, you'll come to Malibu and have a new life with lovers galore."

"Jill, I don't have the strength for lovers," she said.

"Oh, you will. You will. I've never known anyone as full of life as you."

"I get weary sometimes, and I wonder what would happen to Dad if I go first."

I decided to tell my mother what I would do if she died first, thinking such an eventuality might be worrying her.

I said, "I'd talk to Charlie and then I'd get a male nurse. I'd have him come and live with me, Mummy."

The plan visibly set her mind at ease.

Then I said, "But, Mummy, it's more likely with his heart and stroke history that he will go first. You would miss him, you know."

She looked at me, her blue eyes thoughtful. "Oh, yes, I would. I know sometimes I get worn out and exasperated, but I've often thought I wouldn't know what to do without him."

Watching my parents together, I knew that my father would *not* be better off dead. The right decision had been made after all. My parents were very much involved with life, very much alive. I had seen the teasing conversations between them, Daddy shaking his head when I asked if my mother was sweet and she calling him an old bugger. It had ended with Daddy reaching for her hand, pulling himself laboriously to his feet, and getting a kiss. Love was in evidence in the way he carried a chair on which to put her feet so she could take forty winks. Mother, laughing at his attentions. They knew how to live in the moment. They were past masters at that and, yes, love was there.

I could recall visions of my father sitting in the bed of Charlie's truck, watching Charlie and Zuleika build a treehouse on his first visit to Vermont after his stroke. He helped, handing up two-by-fours with his still-strong left hand, very much a part of what was going on, and enjoying such.

Before going to bed that night I studied my father's intelligent eyes. I wondered what made life so worth living for him that he fought so hard for it, dieting, dressing smartly, his desire to be among people and to stay in the best physical condition.

Daddy came to me for a kiss good-night. How easily he did that now, and how easily I gave him the demonstrative affection that had been denied me as a child.

Daddy's stiff-upper-lip Britishness had denied us both the pleasures of kissing and cuddling with me sitting on Daddy's lap, being his little girl. It was out of the question that I should try to flirt or wheedle a favor from him, as I had done with my uncles.

I could not practice my feminine wiles on my father. We had a kind of straightforward, blunt, human-to-human relationship. I cannot understand now why the basic male-femaleness of our personalities were never fully exposed to each other. But they simply weren't. He was my father and I was his daughter and that was that.

For him, I don't think the relationship was unsatisfactory. But to me it was. His maleness did not need anything from a little girl. But every little girl needs something from her father—learning how to relate to the men who would come into her life. I missed those things I saw other little girls share with their fathers. I always dreamed there could be more closeness and I was to witness this basic human simplicity between my daughter Zuleika and her father. Such closeness, cuddling, kissing, stroking, teasing, piggyback rides, pride in her small achievements—nothing too good for her, backing her up against all odds. Unconditional love and oh, how she was cherished. Finally it was part of my life, and I loved watching it. It was almost as if I were a little girl again. I would get as close as I could to all that warmth, all that love, and just try to suck it up, take it inside myself. Lucky Zuleika. Lucky Charlie. To be so uncomplicatedly in love with each other.

But although my father and I had a stilted communication, it did not mean there was not love. While Daddy and I kept our distance, I loved him very much. I have to conclude he loved me. And if he did not tell me so, now that he is mute his eyes express such love and longing to communicate that it squeezes my heart to see so nakedly the emotion that I missed so many years ago. Had I recognized one such loving look when I was still his little girl, how it would have filled up all the empty spaces, all the hurts and the loneliness. Now those looks only tear me apart.

"Good-night, Daddy."

Shortly thereafter I prepared for bed, picturing the two white heads sleeping side by side in the pink, satin-covered twin beds of their room off the suite's sitting room.

As I walked past their door I heard a sudden explosion of sound. It was my father shouting at the top of his lungs, a torrent of uncontrolled, bellowing anger. I heard my mother's soft tones and then there was silence.

Poor Mother, the wrath would surely burst forth when he was home again. My God, how does she stand the constant threat of violent outbursts of anger, the frustration, the sadness? How do they stand it?

I walked impotently to my bedroom, knowing there was nothing I could do. It had all begun long before I was born. The play had started without me in mind. I was a minor player in the drama of their lives. Soon I would be gone, and they both knew it. I would return to Eastbourne after a week in London, but only for a few days. My home was in America. I don't live here anymore.

With these thoughts, I turned out the bedside lamp and lay down to sleep.

55
Adieu

1987

Our little family vacation together was over. This morning we were to leave the Grand Hotel in Eastbourne. I would drop off my parents at their bungalow and then proceed on to London.

I came to the door of Mother's bathroom in the morning and heard the sound of running water.

She said, "Good morning, Jilly. I've been thinking about you a lot."

I closed the door and remained outside. "Oh, did you? What were you thinking?"

"How much I love you. I know I don't always do as I'm told, but I do love you very much."

I was glad the door was closed.

"I love you, too, Mummy. And why should you do as you're told? You do just right."

The door opened and my little mother emerged in a pale-pink cotton nightie, her face pink and white, her hair fluffy, and a lovely smile on her face. She looked as sweet and innocent as a child. I knew I would always remember the way she looked at that moment.

On the way to my parent's home in Seaford, Mummy kept up an excited commentary on familiar landmarks where she and Daddy had visited or walked. Daddy watched her with bright eyes, pointing now and then at a place she might forget. The scenery was wonderful, craggy cliffs of white chalk over the ocean. Downs, rolling hills, fields of lush grass, and dense trees lined the roadway. It was clear my parents had had many happy times since moving from London to Sussex.

They were delighted I was coming to their home. The sky-blue front door, the brilliant hydrangeas in purple, pink, and blue, the lawn green as velvet carpet. A happy, bright home.

Once inside I detected the intangible scent of home, my roots; a scent I knew was discernible only to me. I checked each room, looking at old photographs, Daddy's paintings, the small chair by the fire, the one on which I always sat when I was growing up. I lay on the double bed in the back bedroom. Daddy came in and pulled back the gold candlewick bedspread to show me it was made up and ready to sleep in.

"I'll come back and stay here before I return to America," I said. But he didn't hear me.

I put my head on the pillow inhaling the essence of my beginnings. It was all there in that house, all the familiar smells. My senses stirred. It had been a long time since I had been in touch with those long-lost emotions.

I arose and left by the kitchen door. Daddy was showing Sue the small sunhouse he had built in the garden before his stroke. I kissed and hugged him.

"No," he said, "no."

"I've got to go, Daddy."

He looked infinitely sad.

"I'll see you in a week, after my work in London," I promised.

God, he had thought I was spending the night. A terrible lump stuck in my throat. I hugged Mummy and got into the limousine, waving as we drove slowly away. My parents stood together, waving. As we turned the corner, I saw Daddy lower his head. He was sobbing. I just had time to see Mummy gently turn him toward the house.

London was a continuous round of interviews on television and radio and with the print media, punctuated by quiet dinners in the hotel suite with friends from the past and telephone calls to Charlie back in Los Angeles.

I managed to fulfill my purpose. *Life Wish* quickly became the number-one best-seller in my native islands.

When I did return to Seaford, the small city by the English Channel, Daddy was overjoyed to know I would be staying the night. We spent the evening chatting and watching a bit of television.

My mother had never attempted to hold on to me, but tonight I saw her tentatively reaching out across the years for more time. We recognized each other for the women we were, and we saw the loss. I had felt it for a long time, for years now, but Mummy had not seemed to. This night I saw her yearn.

"Oh, Jilly," she said before kissing me good-night as I lay in bed.

I watched her leave the room. Time was running out.

Jack and Dorothy Ireland were tired the next day, so, like a tourist, I took a bus to the ancient village of Alfriston, founded in the fifteenth century. The houses and shops, some with thatched roofs, were Tudor, the streets narrow and cobblestoned. My English heritage stirred. Sue and I enjoyed a cream tea with scones. We visited the beautiful old church dating back to the early fourteen-hundreds, and we read the many plaques therein. One such bore the names of a man and his wife and the admonition: "You who read this will also die."

The village and its reminders of life, and how quickly it passes, touched me. I was learning acceptance here in the island of my birth. Life is both brief and long.

That evening I went alone to the old redoubt, the fortress that dominates the Eastbourne seaside, to hear a Welsh Guards military band performance. I had not been to a brass-band concert since Mother had taken me as a girl. It was a chilly evening and I pushed back the cold with a glass of burning brandy I had bought at a small bar near the entrance.

I shivered with cold in my jeans and black raincoat. My mind drifted to my first husband, David, and his tender ministrations while I was ill. Now why would that be? Perhaps being surrounded by English people made me think of my English ex-husband, who had been so young during our marriage. I had not seen so many British faces in one place for years.

After intermission, and another brandy, the band struck up a sailor's hornpipe and the audience clapped with enthusiasm. Then "Rule Britannia" and proud, proud singing, accompanied by my tears as I joined in, "Britons, never, never, never shall be slaves."

It would be a long time before I sat again in such a place and listened to such a rendering . . . if ever.

The following day my mother prepared a traditional roast-beef Sunday dinner. Just the three of us. I supplied a bottle of champagne.

After dinner, Daddy took me for an extended walk along the roads, in and out of passages between pretty houses and cottages, their gardens blooming with rhododendrons, roses, and hydrangeas. At one point he walked determinedly up a garden path and knocked on someone's front door. I had no way of knowing who the inhabitants might be. A gentleman opened the door.

"Oh," he said when he saw my father. "Come in then."

"How do you do," I said. "I'm Mr. Ireland's daughter."

"My name is Fred Gale."

My father was pleased that we were meeting. Still not satisfied, he combined *lo lo lo* and *ah ah ah* sounds, insisting on further conversation.

The gentleman's wife appeared. "Have we visitors?" she asked.

Once again I introduced myself. "This is my father. His name is John Ireland."

"We've often wondered who he was," said Mr. Gale.

My father pulled on my sleeve and touched my face. I knew what he wanted but I was reluctant to give him the satisfaction. It was too embarrassing. But Daddy grew more insistent.

I began my party piece. "Mr. and Mrs. Gale, I'm sorry to have to do this, but my father really wants me to introduce myself. My name is Jill Ireland. I live in America."

We chatted for a few minutes before my father said, "Ah ah," indicating I should continue.

"I've written a book. It's called *Life Wish*."

"Ah ah," said Daddy.

I was thoroughly embarrassed to be doing my party piece for two strangers, but they seemed absolutely involved. My father became more insistent. And I spat out as fast as I could: "I'm married to the movie actor Charles Bronson."

"*Ah*," bellowed my father, a self-satisfied sound.

This impressed the Gales. "Charles Bronson, the actor," they said, all round-eyed.

"Quite. Come on, Daddy, we're leaving."

My father was satisfied with this and eagerly left without so much as a backward glance at the amazed Gales.

"I'm sorry we disturbed you," I said as we walked down the garden path.

At home, I recounted the adventure for my mother. I told

her that Mr. Gale showed me a piece of paper on which he had tried to communicate with Daddy using the alphabet. I explained to him that my father's stroke had left him unable to speak, although he understood everything that was said.

"I'll call them later on," Mummy said. "Of course I don't know who he meets on his walks; there's no way he can tell me."

My final three days in England were devoted to a return trip to London with my parents. It was a tonic for them both, especially the evenings when Daddy had gone to bed and Mummy and I in our nightgowns and robes dispatched chocolate sundaes while singing old Ivor Novello–era show tunes.

Too soon, it was time to jet back to my life in America. It was over. Good-bye, good-bye, England. For a while I had entrenched myself in my beginnings. Jill Ireland had come out, helped by old friends and family. I genuinely remembered who I was, what I was, the basic simple me. Now I was returning to what I had become. But I was enriched and strengthened by calling forth the inner me, the base of my personality. I had received such a cornucopia of love, memories, and affection. I had felt truly cherished by my parents.

On the plane from New York to Los Angeles, I still felt different. My American family and life seemed distant, the American Jill remote. I wondered if I would make contact with her, become her again—or if I wanted to.

This trip to the past had been a journey forward, a joining of my two selves. I hoped the fusion would hold when I was back home. I was subtly but definitely changed by the trip.

I remembered the epigram in Alfriston, "You who read this will also die." Okay, but not yet. First, we'll give life a run for its money.

56

Welcome

1987

When I returned to California, I found Jason in his room looking fine, weight just right, eyes bright. I sent out my radar: only good vibrations. I somehow felt back at square one with him. Both Lo Lo and Toy Boy were bathed in golden light for the time being. The light would soon evaporate.

Now it was time to begin moving from Udine Way, my home of twenty years, to the new house in Serra at Malibu, supervising the removal of furniture with my friend and architect-designer King Zimmerman. Only part of our belongings would be transported the twenty-three miles to our new home. The house in Bel Air would continue to be home to Valentine, Katrina, and, occasionally, Jason, until it could be properly prepared for sale.

I pondered how quickly it was all over. It had taken Charlie and me years to furnish and decorate the place. For the first year of our marriage the large sitting room had remained closed, the carved wooden double doors locked, as we slowly assembled paintings and art objects from all over the world. It was the last room finished and now the first to be dismantled. I moved a tapestry-covered magazine box to fill a hole left by an antique, dark wood, country French table that we had purchased in a village in the South of France. Zuleika had not yet been conceived then. How quickly it had all gone. The house would never look the same again. I was lovingly undoing all I had done.

When the van pulled away with several large pieces, I found Charlie sitting in his usual place at the partner's desk in our bedroom, his feet propped on an open drawer. As I lay down on the bed to ease a pain in my lower back, the telephone rang. It was my mother. I was surprised because it was only two days since I had left her. "Dad's had another stroke," she said.

She told me how she had found my father staggering out of the bathroom stark naked and wet, shaking and trembling violently. He fell to the floor thrashing wildly, his arms and legs swinging in an effort to get to his feet.

"Jill, it was dreadful. He was growling and making an awful noise. So violent. He grabbed me, but I couldn't help him up.

"I called a neighbor and the doctor came and injected a sedative."

"How awful, Mummy," I said. "We were wrong to make him have that operation, to live this way."

Mummy said, "Yes, if I knew what to do I would do it. I would . . ."

I stopped her. "Don't say any more."

My mother continued. "He can't walk now, Jill. He's at Three Ways nursing home. At least he knows everyone there. I hope he will be able to walk when he's better. I'm hopeful."

Helpless to do more than sympathize, I made an investment in the future. I invited my mother and father to America for Christmas.

"I don't know, Jill; that's a long way off."

"I know, Mummy, but tell Daddy anyway. Maybe that will encourage him to walk again."

We said good-bye, Jack's two women. My ears were ringing loudly. I felt hard and unemotional; my heart had turned to stone. God, were we all waiting for my father to die so we would be relieved of witnessing his pain? He had fought so savagely to get off the floor, I knew he wasn't ready. He was still strong. Something told me we were not at the end. Not yet. I was to bear witness to more heroic efforts at life.

I telephoned my brother John, who had already spoken to our mother. He sounded hard, too. "I just don't like to see him chipped away at, a piece at a time," John said.

We agreed to meet in Vermont in a week to see the autumn foliage and to be nearer to England.

My back ached and my ears whistled deafeningly. Did I want Daddy to die? No, I wanted him alive, to be near him to kiss and hug, to tease and spoil him. I wanted to love him. While he lived I wanted him to enjoy life.

A day later I was shocked by the state of my own health. I was bleeding vaginally. My menstrual periods had stopped in mid-chemotherapy. The drugs had taken care of that. I made an appointment with my new gynecologist, who told me I must undergo a dilation, curettage, and biopsy in three days.

Now it was important to complete the Serra house by November to accommodate my parents during their holiday visit. It was the only house that did not have steps to climb. It would be the first time in twenty-seven years that my parents and I would celebrate Christmas together. I wanted them in the Serra house to bless it with memories, to make it a home for me.

Two nights before I was due to enter the hospital for my surgery, Charlie and I were at dinner when Valentine entered the room.

"Hi, Val, do you want some dinner?"

Valentine was a bit awkward, almost uneasy. "Well, I *am* hungry."

"Okay, get a place mat and tell the kitchen you're joining us."

My son returned, smiling. Val and Charlie were close; they played golf together several times a week. After dinner I felt mellow and relaxed, the surgery far from my mind, when Val called Charlie from his room, a not uncommon happenstance when they were planning golf games. The conversation was brief. Val called a second time. This time my attention was caught by Charlie's tone. A warning bell rang.

"What is it, Charlie?"

He let me have it straight. "Jason's in jail for drunken driving. He called Val for a thousand dollars' bail."

I just looked at Charlie.

He continued, "Val knew it before dinner, but Jason didn't want you to know."

I also realized Valentine, like me, didn't believe in delivering bad news during dinner. I always tried to keep conversation pleasant while we ate. But dinner was over.

I called Jason's friend Johnny Perkins, with whom he was staying temporarily. He had also received Jason's plea for bail money. Jason had been on his way to see Johnny when he was pulled over by the police in the Bronco, which I had given him permission to drive a few days earlier. Jason had been straight for six months. We had to trust him sometime.

"What should I do, Charlie?"

"I told you, Jason needs a menial job, any job."

"I know, but how do I make him do that?"

"It's too late. He's twenty-five."

"Charlie, you're not answering my question. What shall I do now? Shall I leave him in jail? You always tell me I do the wrong thing."

Charlie didn't want to answer my questions. We held a long three-way conversation on the telephone with Johnny, who was frightened that Jason would freak out if he were sent downtown to a tough jail. I felt we should leave him there, but Charlie said no.

"Get him out," Charlie said, adding that he was through with Jason.

I was numb. My father had had another stroke. I was having surgery in two days, and now Jason was drunk and in jail. Shit. I felt pushed to the wall. My ears were ringing and I knew the spiritual side of me had to be addressed if I were to make it through this new episode of storms. I was still stuck to my rock, but I needed something to stop me from drowning.

57
Fears

1987

I walked along the beach in Malibu, musing about my two males, Lo Lo and Toy Boy, one man dying by inches but fighting like a furious tornado of will to live, the embodiment of "Do not go gentle into that good night."

In contrast was Jason flying so close to the fire, flirting with his destiny, perhaps seducing death to visit him.

Dear God, I have one man dying slowly in England and another in Los Angeles killing himself by inches.

My thoughts flew back to my meeting with Jason on my recent return from England. I searched his face. It was quiet, and within a heartbeat I recognized the withdrawal, the body language that told of much suffering and defeat.

He wore the relaxed pliancy of one who has given up. But what, I asked myself, had he given up? Was it something good or something bad? Oh, I hoped it was not the very essence of himself.

I had shown the same withdrawal the year before I became ill with cancer. It was deep, heavy depression born of a loss of self. I believed my life counted for nothing. Only the lives of my family mattered. I had begun to exist only to serve them, to help them live *their* lives. Mine had no meaning as that of an individual.

I had suffered for a long time, perhaps years, from an identity crisis. The pull between Jill *Ireland* and Jill *Bronson* was confusing, and sometimes saddening.

For instance, when I left telephone messages I found myself stumbling over "Jill Ireland" because to most intents and purposes I was Jill Bronson. The dual personality had become in fact no longer dual. Jill Ireland had been weakening. She simply floated away from me. Never more than at family gatherings when we congregated around a dining table. Everybody had a good time with Charlie as master of ceremonies. And whereas once I had chattered and prattled on, keeping the children amused, introducing new topics for conversation, I now found myself merely going through the formalities.

Jill Ireland would withdraw, leaving Jill Bronson, or at least the flesh that was called Jill Bronson, to eat her dinner making only polite conversation when necessary, and nobody noticed.

Jill Bronson was in a dangerous depression. Jill Ireland knew when to leave a sinking ship. She left town, leaving no forwarding address.

Jill Bronson could not take the abandonment for very long. She decided to throw in the towel and meld completely with this new Ireland-less identity, going so far as to change her first name briefly to Jillian. The first public notice of the change was in an advertisement in the show-business trade papers, *The Hollywood Reporter* and *Daily Variety*, congratulating Mickey Rooney for a particular performance and for his longevity as a star.

The words she chose were: "You are, you have been, and you always will be the greatest. Love, Jillian and Charles Bronson."

The full-page ads completed the anonymity and the

disappearance of Jill Ireland and Jill Bronson. Everyone thought Charlie had taken an ad with his sister or perhaps a daughter—everyone except the person who had placed the ad, me. Whoever that was. Charlie neither approved nor disapproved. He kept his silence.

It was a deep cry of despair, gone unheard, as I threw in the towel. Jillian Bronson did not exist; never existed. It was simply abject depression that encouraged me to put Jillian in the place of those Bronson and Ireland women—a sort of Stepford Wife.

Now I recognized the same disillusioned sadness, the quiet acceptance, in Jason.

How it pained me to know there was nothing I could do. Oh, the ineffable sadness in those eyes as they looked at me, confused and tormented, accepting their fate. No fight. No source. Just withdrawn acceptance. Depression.

It had taken a close brush with death for me to fight back. When this creature Jillian Bronson became ill, Jill Ireland arrived pronto, took over the proceedings, moved back in, never to depart again.

The essence of me was all inside Jill Ireland and when I withdrew her essence, only an empty, resigned body inhabited that space. If it hadn't been for the cancer, who knows what would have happened.

I wondered what Jason needed to bring back his essence, and still resist his dangerous, dark energy. Maybe it would take a catastrophe as profound as mine to make him whole. I hoped not.

I loved the essence of Jason and I knew how impoverished and meaningless his life must seem without it.

The symbiosis with him became immediately apparent. I experienced an inexplicable fear and sadness. Serious, real fear—the sort accompanied by fluttery sensations of disquiet that start in the diaphragm. This was not good for me. Things that lay buried all day, kept at bay by daylight and the day's activity, were released while I slept, freed from the prison I had built for them deep inside my brain, a strong, complicated prison in a never-visited area. These fears did not escape easily; they only broke loose and made their presence felt by entering my dreams.

They betrayed their presence just as I entered that place between sleep and awakening. Then the subtle but definite tapping at my consciousness started. *We're here. Help.* Each morning I awakened with the fears telling me they were trying to dig their way out before I was fully conscious and able to push them back.

"Help us. Help us."

Each insidious cry made me more nauseated and full of dread. I couldn't quite believe this. I could always control my fears, or at least understand them enough to live with them. But this was terrible, this unknown horror. The intensity stayed with me for about sixty seconds. Any longer I couldn't stand. As it was, I was afraid I was becoming unstable. My flight from these fears was making my dance of life, my trip to remission, dazzlingly bright and exhausting. I was running too hard. I had to stop.

One morning I awoke and could barely get out of bed. My left leg wouldn't straighten out to touch the floor. Putting on my underwear was almost impossible. I considered going out without underpants, but after stepping into them as they lay on the floor and maneuvering for five minutes, I managed with the aid of the crook of an umbrella to hike them high enough up my legs to get them into place.

My surgeon Mitchell Karlan made an appointment for me with a radiologist. I caught myself up short as I sat in an immodest cotton gown on the cold steel of the X-ray table. I looked down at my white-cotton socks and became aware of a feeling of security. It suffused my body, a sensation I imagined not unlike that of an infant when it is full of warm milk. I felt secure. When I recognized the emotion, I broke out in goose bumps. I realized it was the familiar surroundings of a doctor's office where everything was being taken care of. If indeed I was seriously ill, I would probably be put to bed, given more tests. People would step in to take over for me. Ye gods, was I welcoming illness as a way out from under?

No. No. No. I didn't want it. I would not have it. This sneak attack on my psyche was from that familiar monster that lurked within my brain, unable to gain ground by its previous tactics of terror. It was now seducing me into embracing comfortable dependence in the guise of soft, soothing voices, sympathetic eyes, a gentle hand on the shoulder applied with sincere concern, white-coated assistants helping me to lie comfortably on the table.

Absolutely not, Jill Ireland! I had too much to do.

We had to be moved into the Serra house by the week of December seventh, when my parents were to arrive. The little guest cottage by the pool was ready for them. I was forcing D-day. I had to be well, have my health sorted out in the next two weeks so I could care for and nurture my mother and father. They needed it. Then there was Christmas, the usual hurly-burly of gift buying, decorations, and all the rest.

I would be ready, and so would the Serra house.

The X ray showed a bulging disc and I was in the grip of a sciatic nerve attack. I buckled down and healed on schedule.

58

Resolve

1987

One day I came into the Bel Air house to find Jason cooking in the kitchen. Sitting at the table was a man. The blood hit the top of my head. I stood staring in rage.

I had told Jason the previous day that he was to have no visitors without permission. And here he was, only one day later, entertaining, cooking for a stranger.

I pointed a finger at the man and said, "You! Get out. Now!"

Then I turned furious eyes on my son.

"And you, Jason, should contact your natural mother and talk to *her*. Maybe she can straighten you out. I've done all I can."

At the mention of his birth mother, Jason blew up. He clenched his fists and his eyes filled with tears. He walked out of the kitchen and into the back pantry. I followed him. "I mean it, Jason. I think you should find your mother. Maybe it will help. I'm burned out."

"I don't want to talk about it," he said.

This scene took place in February of 1987. Now it was

November of that year and we had come a long way. Now Jason was ready. He wanted to see his natural mother.

I telephoned George Henderson, the lawyer who had arranged the adoption twenty-five years earlier. Henderson said it was possible to contact the aunt with whom Jason's mother was living at the time of the adoption. He suggested Jason come to his office for whatever information was available in his files.

As it turned out, Henderson was full of misinformation.

Jason, on a high about meeting the woman who bore him, met with Henderson the next day. The lawyer gave him photographs of his birth mother taken before he was born. He had found a means of reaching her and said she would telephone him the following day.

"Vicky was gorgeous," Henderson told me on the telephone. "But she had serious problems."

He tried to talk me out of contacting her. He said Jason's grandmother had been a prostitute, that Vicky had been hospitalized for psychiatric reasons several times; that she hadn't seen her own father since she was fourteen. He added that Vicky was a part-time model and supermarket checker when Jason was born.

A day later I heard from Jason. His voice was choked and I could hear muffled sobs. "Mom, I just came back from seeing Henderson," he said. "I just see darkness and blackness. I can't handle hearing all that stuff about my mother. I feel sick, seriously, seriously sick."

My heart pounded. I felt the responsibility. I'd done it. It had been my idea to contact his mother. A friend of mine said I had been trying to play God. No. I only followed my instincts. I had been guided by love, hadn't I? Hadn't I?

"Come here to the beach, Jason," I said.

"I can't."

"Why not?"

"It's raining and it's cold."

Jason sounded as if he were losing it.

"Jason, is Lisa there with you?"

"Yes."

"Put her on."

A young, frightened, and breathless voice said, "Yes?"

"Lisa, bring him here. You can both stay overnight."

Jason returned to the phone. "I'm coping. This is the hardest blow I've ever had. But I want to handle it with strength."

"Jason, the strongest blow you received is the day Vicky gave you away. You can handle a blow you know about, the one you see and feel. But you can't cope with a wound you never knew you received—you just keep bleeding internally until you discover the source, or it kills you."

"But Mom, I'm so scared of what I'll discover."

I assured him that contacting his birth mother would be a meaningful step in his life.

"Mom, my instincts tell me this is going to be the key that opens my door. I didn't like what the lawyer told me. My God, could I have inherited her background? I don't want to be like her. It bothers me to think that is the way I am. At least I didn't try to put a gun to my head like she did.

"Did you know that when I was a little kid she called Henderson's office and said she wanted to see and talk to me or else she would kidnap me? And when I was eighteen she tried to get to me. She said she needed to be with me."

As he said this, I saw a flash, an image. Time receded. Vicky and Jason fused in my mind. The infant was craved by the mother. I sensed the decision to offer him for adoption had ruined her life. She regretted. Was I the only one who didn't regret?

"God, Jason," I said, "if she had seen you at eighteen she would have had quite a surprise."

My remark was rewarded by Jason's hearty, juicy chuckle. As he thought it over the chuckle deepened into the familiar rich belly laugh.

"You're right, Mom. She'd have wondered what hit her.

She doesn't know how lucky she was not to have found me."

"Maybe it would have been the right thing," I said. "Perhaps she was picking up your distress signals. Maybe she was responding. She knew you needed her. Maybe that would have stopped you. Who knows?"

We both fell silent. Then Jason said, "Mom, I feel sorry for her. I want to talk to her the way you talk to me, you know? Her life's a mess."

Now I felt alarm.

"Don't get sucked into that," I said.

I remembered Henderson's words, spoken rather sardonically but nevertheless, I recalled his saying a reunion might resurrect them both. I hoped such a meeting would finally help Jason stand up alone. If we helped Vicky, that would be great. After all, I owed her a debt. And to paraphrase Jason so many years earlier, we should thank her for not having an abortion.

I was twice tied into these events. I had chosen to become Jason's mother; I knew I would not give up a single day of that little boy's childhood to unburden myself of the sadness and pain he brought me later in his life.

A few days later Jason saw Vicky.

59
Reunion

Kier entered the restaurant. The intoxicating, pungent aroma of spicy food invaded his nostrils, but he disregarded all of this.

Kier drove Jason straight across the room and into her arms.

She gasped when she saw him.

Kier allowed himself to meld, becoming one with his mother. He felt himself leaving Jason, slipping effortlessly, timelessly into the empty place under his mother's heart.

With a sigh, he settled in.

60
Family Ties

1987

Jason's voice on the telephone was different. I heard a lot of defense and toughness. He sounded hard, really hard, not put-on tough-guy stuff.

He had just seen Vicky.

"She told me, Mom, my father's family is Mafia and that I had three brothers. One of them died.

"All kinds of weird things, but I had to believe her. It all fits. She told me my birth father was a heroin addict who died of an overdose after I was born. He had already left her before I was born to go back to his own wife and kids when they all lived in Detroit. She moved out here to have me. Vicky was never married to my father, and the other three boys had different fathers, Mom. I have two half brothers living here in Los Angeles someplace right now.

"Vicky said she couldn't keep me *and* my older three brothers. She was broke and needed money for food and medical care when she was pregnant with me. She thought I would have a better life if another family adopted me."

Jason went on to say that Vicky had been ill through

much of her pregnancy. From the very beginning of the adoption proceedings, she knew that David and Jill McCallum were adopting her infant. She told Jason she had been informed that the young English couple would return to the British Isles and that she would never hear about or see her baby again. But when David starred in the TV series "The Man from U.N.C.L.E.," and I began appearing in American films and TV, Vicky followed our careers, trying at irregular intervals to contact Jason through the attorney George Henderson.

Vicky told Jason that she had been unable to handle the loss of the baby she gave away. She had met the next-door neighbor of the McCallums and begged her to take a photograph of Jason, but the woman refused.

Vicky's story was filled with heartbreak, tragedy, death, and drugs, all of which profoundly disturbed Jason.

Now *I* understood so much more. God, had I been unequipped to rear this child, this son of a Mafia drug dealer. His mother and I twisted his fate.

Vicky told Jason that ever since his birth she had been trying to see him, that she had never given up. George Henderson did not tell the young English couple about Vicky's psychological problems.

She told Jason, "If your father's family knew about you, they would take you. They are Mafia, your uncles."

My head reeled. I remembered Henderson's words of seven years earlier when I requested help in finding Jason's mother. At that time I told him about Jason's wildness and drug addiction.

Henderson said he was sorry about the problems, but that Vicky was a mixed-up, troubled woman. And he suggested, "I wouldn't open that can of worms."

It appears that after the adoption Henderson shielded me from Jason's birth mother, discouraging her telephone calls, never relaying messages, and always telling her it would not be possible to see Jason, that she should leave us alone.

But I wonder now if it would not have been better had Jason and Vicky met before it was too late. Perhaps Vicky and I should have met before the adoption, and it might well have been better if Vicky had received counseling and emotional support during and after her decision.

It is natural to think of the birth mother as out of the picture once the adoption papers are signed and the baby handed over. But because of the nature of the basic relationship between mother and child, the natural mother will always be in the picture somehow, somewhere.

Now, twenty-five years later, Vicky and I were going to have the conversation we needed and craved for so long. I only hoped that better-late-than-never would be applicable.

I was surer than ever that Jason had been born an addict, if not in his chemistry, in his soul.

He himself felt it to be so.

"It was floating around in my system," Jason said. "All it needed was the trigger. The Ritalin did that. That was the trigger."

Vicky told him how one of his half brothers had saved her from being raped. He chased her assailant and stopped a bullet that struck him in the head. He lived only one more year.

Jason said Vicky told him she had taken drugs and that her health was not good. That and the news his father died of an overdose must have come as the shock of all time to Jason, who had been told all along that his birth father was an architect, a married man leading a conservative life—the father of two children. For those specious reasons his mother had never informed his father of Jason's birth. The picture was changing rapidly for Jason and me.

It seemed Vicky harbored terrible resentment toward me, believing I had kept Jason from her. God, David and I thought we had legally adopted a baby, paid for it, cared for it. Surely, that was what I had the right to do. She knew I had had cancer and had seen me on a TV show talking about it. She told Jason she had screamed at the TV set, "You bitch! I'll get you, you bitch!"

Oh, Vicky, I said to no one, I didn't ever want to steal your child. I only wanted to mother one.

But this was not all. We had to learn more. Jason said Vicky told him she had thrown herself down a flight of stairs to try to kill the baby she was carrying.

He said, "I've always known it. It was in the darkness, darkness, darkness. She tried to kill me."

Jason and I spoke quietly for a few moments. Then each of us, deep in our own thoughts, bid one another good-night. I couldn't get it out of my mind that this woman who carried Jason's heritage, who had to be in many respects much like him, hated me. It hurt. I didn't hate her. And it mattered to me that she know that.

The thought of Vicky stayed with me. I was also a little frightened to have aroused such hostility. I couldn't let it rest.

Some days later, with a nervous, fluttery stomach and trembling arms, I dialed her number. I was scared.

A surprisingly childlike voice answered with a tremulous, "Hello."

In my most measured tones I said, "Hello, Vicky, this is Jill. Do you know who I am?"

"My God, of course I know who you are. I've wanted to talk to you. Why didn't you answer my messages?"

"I haven't received any messages. But we're talking now. It's good to hear your voice after all these years. I can't tell you how many times I've thought of you and wanted to speak to you."

She sounded as if she were crying. "I'm so nervous," she said. "I get into trouble wording things. They come out wrong."

"That's all right, Vicky. Jason does that too."

"Oh, my God," she said. "Jason. When I met him I went from hell to heaven. Since I met Jason I've tried crystal, which is black cocaine. My suggestion to you is, try it. It will make you feel better."

The hair on the back of my neck began to rise.

"You know I hated you," she continued. "I couldn't understand why you wouldn't let me see him. I called every year on his birthday."

"I didn't know that," I said quietly.

As we spoke, I found in spite of my former anxiety and the remark about cocaine, that I began to like this woman.

She said, "I sent a telegram to George Henderson because my son's life is at stake. I'm frightened he may die like one of my other boys, and I couldn't bear to go through that again. You know, when I met Jason he kept holding me. He said his life was like a puzzle. If he wants to go into a clinic I will go with him. I will do anything. I'm so scared he will die."

In a voice trembling with fear, Vicky said, "He doesn't need to see me anymore, Jill. All I want is for him to let me give him anything I can and for him to be okay. God, he's beautiful. It's not just his looks, it's inside him. You know, Jill, I brought all the love for all my children with me when I met him. I love him so much I don't care if I die, but I want him to live. He's so like his father. I was blown away when he told me about the heroin, his addictions."

Vicky was well informed. She quoted statistics. At one point she sounded like me when she said, "Why do I get more upset than other people? I can't stop thinking about it. That's all I do. Jason should be on Antabuse. Alcohol causes most problems. The highest percentage of people in the county jail are involved with crimes related to alcohol. Make him give you a urine sample every day. When they're straight they will give you urine."

I tried to comfort her. "But Vicky, he's straight now."

She was inconsolable: "His grandfather was an alcoholic. I never saw him after I was fourteen. I think you've been through hell with him, Jill. I understand because I was there with the son I lost. I want to put him together for you. Oh, my God, don't you understand, he could die like that."

I found it hard to keep up with the flow of conversation from this disembodied voice. Once I called her Jason's mother.

She responded vehemently. "No, I'm not. Please don't call me that. It hurts me. You're his mother."

"Vicky," I said, "it just so happens that this person has two mothers because you never cut the cord."

As the conversation went on we spoke like two mothers. I told her how when Valentine was born I had told Jason that Val was his baby.

"I did that with my boys," she said.

We laughed and exchanged stories of our children's babyhood and childhood. She told me of her granddaughter and how beautiful she was.

And then it was time to wind it up. I told Vicky I had enjoyed speaking with her. I promised I would call if there were ever a problem with Jason. We said good-bye like two old friends.

I hung up the phone. When I told Charlie I had called her, he asked, "Why?"

"She's Jason's flesh and blood. I did it for me, not Jason," I said. "I had to share the pain. It was the first time in twenty-five years that I felt I wasn't alone with him, that someone else loved him as much as I did. I was sharing the pain, Charlie."

61
Annie

1987

I said, "Hera?"

She said, "No. I'm Annie."

She was standing pathetically forlorn at the foot of the staircase in the Bel Air house.

I looked at her narrow face, hopelessly thin body, the pretty, soft brown hair, the youth, and I knew I was looking death in the eye, a living death that would not ever see thirty.

There were open sores at the corners of her mouth, on her legs, arms, and cheeks. Her eyes were haunted. It was a bitterly cold November day for California and she was shivering. She looked to be no more than eighteen, although in fact she was twenty-three, quite old for a street prostitute.

She scammed me.

I helped her.

Annie said her mother had died two days earlier in Montreal of a heart attack. She said she had leukemia. She said her pimp, Winston, would not let her back in the house unless she gave him one hundred and forty dollars. She told me she robbed people on the street, said she hadn't slept for three days. She showed me her feet, bare skin, red and raw from walking.

I held her in my arms. She cried. She may have been lying, but her lies and her need of them broke my heart.

What pitiful walking debris remained of the profit to be made from drugs.

I gave her all the money in my purse; then I fed her. I recognized the body language, the rubbing of her legs, the shifting restlessness. I saw it and I knew.

After she left, I telephoned Jason.

I said, "A friend of yours was here. She said she had been staying with you in this house some time ago and she was looking for some of her clothes. But she was really looking for you, Jason. She was desperate, so I gave her some money, a warm sweater, and a jacket."

Jason groaned, "Oh, no, Mom. No. Not her. You gave it to the wrong one. She's a con artist."

"I don't care, Jason. I couldn't bear it. It was so sad."

Jason's voice became firm. "Mom, stop it. It wasn't me. It's not me. I'm all right. I don't want you giving money to every little drug addict who comes to the door. It's not me."

"Okay," I said. I told him I loved him and hung up.

But I knew for the rest of my life I would always recognize the pain and suffering of the children afflicted with the disease called drug addiction.

In retrospect, I wonder how and why I let it continue, the procession of pimps, prostitutes, pushers, deadbeats, thieves, and possibly worse, that at one time or another used Jason's quarters in our home as a clubhouse.

I had blinded myself and simply treated them as his friends, so anxious was I to have my son safe under my roof. I was prepared at almost any cost to put up with the flotsam he dragged into our home.

As I came to know some of them so intimately, my heart was dragged into the relationships and I found myself identifying with their tragedies and the sorrow they had brought their families.

Had it not been for Jason's room, many of those people would have been sleeping in the streets.

62
Isolation

1987

Only two weeks before Christmas my parents arrived from Eastbourne for the holidays and to welcome in 1988.

Miracle of miracles, the Serra house was ready and my mother and father took up residence in the sunny guest house. The main residence was still in a state of flux, but Charlie, Zuleika, and I had moved in to celebrate our first Christmas in our new home.

The family gathered for the traditional feast songs and gift giving. Charlie's splendid, towering tree was impressively decorated, a yearly chore in which he took rightful pride. Our dogs, Cassie, my faithful German shepherd, and Celia, our great white kuvasz, had settled in as had our three cats.

My parents enjoyed the change of scenery and the pleasant, clement weather. Despite his most recent stroke, Daddy did not seem much changed. My mother, however, continued to look a bit weary.

Shortly after celebrating the New Year, I said to my father, "Do you know what I think? In your next life, Dad, you won't have any problems. You've had enough in this one."

Gently, lovingly, his face soft, he looked at me. His eyes searched mine.

"Ah," he said, so quietly.

"Really, Dad, in your next life I know you won't have any problems."

He was struggling with strong emotions, and in the fight a huge gasp escaped.

"It's true, Dad."

I held him, put my cheek against his, and spoke carefully into his ear. "You've been brave and you've been strong. I think you are wonderful."

He began to weep and I fought my own feelings so that I could say clearly, "I am proud of you, Dad. I am very proud of you."

He looked at me, shook his head, then cupped my face with his hand. He looked right into me. I saw the man emerge from the travesty. Then he brushed his hair back and regained control. I patted him, pulled away, and went back to my chair.

It had been a different evening. The four of us, Charlie, my mother, Daddy, and I, had had dinner together, my mother doing most of the talking, prattling on about England, her rates and taxes and the lot of old people. She looked pretty this night, her white hair shining in the light, matching the white collar that framed her face. She wore the pink sweater my father had given her for Christmas.

Daddy was quiet and thoughtful through the meal, not attempting to cup his ear to try to catch parts of the conversation. After dinner we went into the billiard room. Charlie stood looking at the table. There was no one to give him a game this evening. Then, to my surprise, my father selected a cue and indicated tentatively, almost shyly, that he wanted to try.

I became anxious, knowing how protective Charlie was of his table.

"Let him try, Charlie, please," I said. "If he tears the cloth I will replace it. Let him try."

"He won't be able to do it," Charlie said.

"But he wants to and it's the first time he's ever shown interest in anything like this. Please let him try."

I fetched the wooden cue bridge for my father and put it on the table. Then I held my breath as Daddy, balancing precariously with a quavering left hand, put the long stick in the middle groove of the bridge. He gently tapped the white cue ball. It rolled two inches.

I applauded. Then it was Charlie's turn. With a sharp *crack* he separated the balls and they flew in all directions on the table.

He turned to my father and said, "Jack, can you make a bridge with your fist, like this?"

He placed the knuckles on his left hand on the table and slid the cue back and forward over them.

"He can't," I hissed. "His arm is paralyzed."

"I know," said Charlie, "but I thought maybe he could lay it on the table."

"Charlie, he can't move his arm."

Daddy hit a few more balls, each one a little more firmly. Then he finally gave up, shaking his head in disgust.

Charlie began clearing the balls from the table, pocketing one after another. *Crack. Crack. Crack.*

"Just a minute," I said. "Hold on. Don't you think for this game you should play with your left hand only. It's only fair after all."

Charlie took the cue in his left hand and began tapping the balls.

"It's not easy," he said. "And I'm taller than your father, which gives me an advantage. I think his last stroke has made his left arm weaker."

Soon Charlie had pocketed all the balls and we retired to the sitting room.

There was a fire blazing in the hearth. My mother began chatting about a club for stroke victims to which my father belonged. She said most of the members were more physically handicapped than Daddy, in wheelchairs and on crutches. But all of them managed to communicate somehow, no matter how long it took them to get the words out.

She said, "Jack's the only one who has completely lost the ability to communicate."

Charlie, knowing Daddy could sing, asked my mother if my father had tried to sing instead of speak words.

In the flickering firelight Daddy watched earnestly.

I explained tensely to Charlie, "The songs are locked in his memory. He sings only old songs he used to know. You can't teach him new ones, and even then the words aren't really clear."

"They used to be," said Charlie.

I stood up and approached my father. "Watch this," I said to Charlie.

"Dad," I said in a loud, clear voice. "What's that song we sing about dickie birds?"

He looked at me, nonplussed.

"You know, Daddy, the ones about dickie birds on the sea."

He sat quietly, intensely concentrating, trying to remember the song, every fiber in his being straining. It was clear he wasn't going to get it, so I began to sing.

Then his face cleared. He joined in. "Poor little dickie birds out on the sea. Poor little dickie birds, oh, dear me."

As he sang, I backed away from him and let my voice soften and fade away, miming vigorously so he still thought I was singing. But he was singing alone.

Now Charlie could hear how the words sounded. They weren't words at all, really, more the rhythm of word. My father's eyes began to look insecure and his voice faltered, so

I joined my voice with his loudly, energetically, and we finished the song together.

"Jill," my mother prompted. "See if he still remembers 'The Red, Red Robin.'"

I started: "When the red, red robin comes bob-bob-bobbin' along."

He remembered and joined in. I let my voice fade again and he sang alone, "Cheer up, cheer up, you sleepy head. Get up, get up, get out of bed."

He was suddenly in the grip of an emotion. He stopped, covering his mouth with his hand and bowing his head, shaking it. He wept, sobbing.

I had touched the inner nerve. I had made him feel the pain that he had numbed. Now it came up and grabbed us both by our throats, the full horrible reality of his situation.

It was almost as if I heard a thin line from space, "Oh, Jill, you too. You've had problems too."

His face seemed to lose the years. His image dissolved in my eyes. He looked twenty years younger and it was the old Daddy sitting with me, not the cute clown he had become. The brave, cute clown.

We were speaking to each other, words without words. I wondered why I did it. Why did I cup my hands, fill them to the brim with that pain? Why did I disturb it? Would it have been better to leave it alone, as they say, let sleeping dogs lie? I know as long as I live I will never forget looking into the soul of that man and sharing the lonely sadness of his existence just for a few moments.

I stepped forward and sang loud and clear, my voice echoing up into the high Spanish ceiling and down the hallways. But Daddy could not continue. He remembered. I knew he did. It was then that I put my arms around Florence Ireland's youngest son, little Jack Ireland. How it would have hurt her to see him this way, and Frederick Ireland, old at forty. How would he have felt to see his Jack now, to know of his life of suffering?

I hoped Frederick knew his granddaughter cared. I sat in the chair next to my father. He touched my face so tenderly. My heart was swollen with emotion. I looked deep into him and shared the full enormity of my father's prison. I understood how he had to play the clown, to be cute, to laugh. The void was immense. For Jack there was no way out, the journey endless. His ticket was going the whole way. I saw the man within and it was tragic.

63

Dorothy's Advice

1988

"Jill," said my mother, straightening her back and tucking in her chin, as was her custom when she was about to impart something of uneasy significance. "When you wish things for Zuleika, wish her only health and happiness. That is all she really needs. I sometimes feel a little uncomfortable about all the wishing and daydreaming I did long before you were born.

"When I was a little girl I used to go into a back room with my dolls and daydream and wish for all the things that eventually happened to you. I was most romantic and played with my dolls, very much like Snow White singing 'Some day my prince will come.' Though of course I hadn't seen the film because it hadn't been made yet.

"I've often thought you ended up living my dream. It wasn't your dream at all. Mothers should be careful what they dream about and what they think they want, because it might come true in the next generation."

Her words echoed what I had been thinking for some time—that I had been living out my mother's fantasies.

We were rattling along Lincoln Boulevard in my old Corvette Stingray. I looked at my mother in her pale dusty-rose cotton turtleneck and black slacks, her foot braced against the floorboard. The colorful, painted Mexican walking stick that had been mine during my long siege with broken legs was pushed between her knees.

She appeared concerned.

"Don't worry, Mother, it wasn't a bad dream."

"Oh, no," she said. "It wasn't. But all the same, when you wish for Zuleika, wish only for her health and happiness."

64
Waves

1988

It was January, a new year, and I was awakened by a call from my beach-house neighbors. Southern California was in the midst of a horrendous high tide with towering waves pounding the coastline from Mexico to Santa Barbara. My little house was not immune. The seething brine was buffeting over the steps leading up from the sand to my downstairs bedroom.

"You'd better come quickly, Jill," my neighbors said.

I grabbed Cassie and off we went for the five-minute drive from the Serra house to the beach house.

It was a beautiful, sparkling day. The terrible winds that had blown all night erased all traces of clouds and smog. The air was crystal pure and clean. The sea boiled furiously.

My house was a hive of activity. The neighbors were clustered on their verandas. Bob Patten, my neighbor, had entered my bedroom through the shattered remains of the window beside my four-poster bed where a wave had crashed.

The sea roared, hissed, and writhed in paroxysms of fury.

In spite of my horror I found it terribly exciting. Great black walls of water gathered on the horizon and came rolling toward where I stood by the sopping bed. I stared at them as they came closer and closer, excitement mounting within me. Then the tips of their black walls would turn over in contemptuous snarls of white foam.

I found myself daring them, saying, "Come on, come on, smash into the house. C'mon."

Then with a resounding crash, Mother Nature hurled herself on my home. It shuddered from the blow. A cacophony of sound surrounded me. Another window shattered and water, sand, and glass engulfed the room.

My emotions of the past eight weeks were suddenly, massively mimicked, put into tiny perspective by nature.

The huge waves raced in, each bigger than the last, destroying the tranquil beach. The sand, which my house had been resting on, was washed away, exposing enormous boulders placed there by the previous owner to protect the supports and underside of the house. The advancing monsters carried all sorts of debris, chairs, logs, even a telephone pole.

I stayed in the downstairs room. The tide had turned and was beginning to ebb, but the water still poured through my broken windows. My area rugs were washed up against the back wall.

My stepson Tony and two carpenters, who had been working at the Serra house, arrived and carried my furniture, TV set, and books—everything they could lift—up to the safety of the garage. I sat with Cassie on my four-poster with water sloshing around, fascinated by nature's hysterics.

Mother Nature, to whom I had been so closely tied the past few days, finally had had it with me.

"You think you've had problems?" she seemed to say to me. "Well, watch this. I can destroy your carefully put-together world, your piles of books, meticulously placed family photographs, and ornaments with one flick of my wrist."

Oh, she was in raging form. I watched her coming, curling, thundering on the horizon, snarling at me, her lips foaming in contempt as she approached. A mountain of black water once again battered against the house.

Cassie and I, wide-eyed, backed against the headboard of the bed and stood our ground. But this time she didn't reach us. Perhaps she didn't want to. Her temper had abated.

Mother Nature had mirrored my emotions of anger. Now, after the smart slap on the wrist she had delivered, she calmed down and was sparkling beautifully, like a brilliant woman at a banquet, dressed in her best jewels, clear-eyed and innocent looking.

The horizon became as still as a millpond. The storm was over. All that remained was to clean up after her magnificent show of histrionics.

65

The Circle Completed

1988

For some reason I wanted to be in my Stingray, the car in which I had reared my children. The car in which Jason had loved to ride all those years ago.

I was coming full circle back to the beginning, back twenty-five years. I drove from the beach along the Pacific Coast Highway, up Sunset Boulevard, past the old house in Bel Air, on through Beverly Hills, past Benedict Canyon where I lived when Jason was born, on up to the Mirabelle restaurant on the Sunset Strip. I parked the Corvette, took a long look at my eyes in the driving mirror to see who was inside looking out. The expression was quiet, but there were deep circles beneath them. I powdered my nose and then thought to myself, It won't make any difference to her if your nose is shiny.

I walked into the Mirabelle. As I crossed the threshold, a dark-haired woman with a soft aura surrounding her and with a kind, gentle face approached me with her arms out.

We embraced and I stood back and looked in her eyes.

I spoke to her: "He looks just like you."

She smiled nervously.

"I don't know if they have a table here," she said.

"I've got to pee," I said.

Vicky seemed to know the restaurant and she led me around to the ladies' room. As I entered, I said, not expecting an answer: "Have you been here before?"

I received a tremulous smile and I closed the door and went in. I stood before the mirror for a few moments composing myself. We had met after all those years.

I was going to have lunch with the mother of my son.

I washed my hands and returned to her. We went to an outside table on the patio and sat beneath a beige-green umbrella overlooking the boulevard.

She said, "I don't know why, but I feel like I know you."

"You do know me," I said. "And I know you."

"No, you don't," she said, smiling.

"Yes, I do. Because, you see I *know* Jason."

I found myself staring at the face of the woman who had carried my child. I tried hard to control it, not wanting to embarrass her. But I could not stop. Never again in the future would I be so struck as I was at that moment by the family resemblance. He had her face, the bone structure, her blue eyes, dark blue with long, straight lashes, her thick, luxuriant hair and finely etched dark brows.

They had the same pallor and yet there was a soft glow to the skin. I also noted they both bit their fingernails to the quick. When she asked if she could smoke, and then lit up a long, thin cigarette, in the way she dragged the smoke into her lungs and tilted her head, I again saw my son. And because I saw my son, I felt a surge of affection, a feeling more akin to love than I was comfortable with or knew how to deal with.

This woman was family. For twenty-five years I had taken care of and loved so desperately the fruit of her womb. And now, at last, there was someone with whom to share that love, someone who loved him as much as I did.

"Jason's got a job," I said, giving her the best gift immediately.

I could see she was glad, really glad.

"He's working in a lunch shop making sandwiches, and on his days off he's working on a construction site with a friend."

Oh, it was wonderful to show these treasures to someone who would really appreciate them. Our drug-addicted son had a job. Not one but two. He was straight.

We ordered salads for lunch. I noticed her hands were shaking. She told me she had waited so long to see Jason, and when he had walked into the restaurant where they had met for the first time, she floated with happiness. Jason said he had needed to hold her and she had certainly needed to hold him, she said.

"Oh, he is so beautiful," Vicky said.

I agreed.

The pain that had been lodged in my heart for so many years was slowly dissolving.

During the next four hours I reached out and communicated with her and Vicky did the same. She showed me photographs of her other three sons, of the youngest who had the same mischievous gleam in his face that Jason could show, and the oldest, handsome, ethereal, the one who had presented her with a beautiful little granddaughter. And the son who had died tragically. When I saw the photograph of him I gasped. He was arresting, really good-looking, much more so than Jason. And yet there was such a similarity, and the noses were identical.

Tears filled my eyes as I looked at the picture and I saw Vicky controlling herself. He had been her passion, the one she confessed she loved the most.

Vicky looked at me and said, "You know, I feel a little better about it all since I met Jason. I gave him my boy's ring, you know."

I said I did.

The air was turning cooler. Vicky had picked at her fruit salad. I sensed she had ordered only it out of shyness and I insisted she eat fish, protein, I suggested, to adjust her chemistry.

"It's bad," I told her, "to eat only fruit. It will send your blood sugar up and then plummeting down, leaving you depressed and tired."

She submitted and I ordered some broiled fish and vegetables and I watched, gratified, as happily as I had watched Jason eat his spaghetti that night two years earlier. I wanted her to be nourished.

When it grew too cold for us to sit longer on the patio, I asked how she had arrived at the restaurant. Vicky had taken a taxi.

I offered to drive her home and we repaired like two girlfriends to the elderly Stingray. By now, Vicky, clad only in black jeans, a thin cotton shirt, and black cotton sweater around her shoulders, was trembling with cold. I pulled a bulky blue pullover out of the back of the car and gave it to her.

"Here, keep yourself warm," I said.

She tucked it around herself and placed her hands beneath it, saying, "I'll just warm my hands."

I was glad I had insisted she eat the fish.

How strange it was. Here I was driving Jason's mother home in the car in which he had so often ridden, this woman who had yearned for him for so many years. We made off down Sunset Boulevard, passing Hillside Avenue, the street where, by turning our heads to the left we could see, nestled against the hill, the white-stucco Spanish-Mediterranean house that Jason had lived in until he was five.

"I knew your next-door neighbor when you lived there. I tried to get his wife to lean over the wall and take a picture of him, I was so desperate to see him. But she wouldn't. You know I was in love with David. I nearly met him once when he was recording at RCA one afternoon.

"I told George Henderson, the lawyer, I was going to do this and he asked me not to. He said, 'For the sake of the boy, Vicky. For the sake of the boy.' And even though I was so in love with David, I said, 'For the sake of the boy, I won't.'"

Her words were a stream of consciousness.

"You see," she said, as we proceeded along Sunset and down onto Hollywood Boulevard, "when I lost Jason, all the love I had for him I projected onto David. That seems crazy now, but that's the way it was. I was very angry with you when you left him and married Charles Bronson. You see, I wanted David McCallum to raise my son."

This was all an old story to me. I'd heard it before from the lawyer. But it was odd hearing it firsthand. I remember how frightened I'd been that Vicky would try to kidnap Jason. And almost as if she read my mind, she said, "I didn't want to kidnap him or anything. I just wanted to look at him.

"You know, when he was born I was worried because his father was a drug addict. I was afraid he wouldn't have all his fingers and toes. But he's perfect. He was perfect, wasn't he? So beautiful."

By now we were in the Hollywood area. The neighborhoods were getting seedier and seedier. I saw a homeless, gray-bearded man with a bedroll sorting through a garbage can, eating scraps. We went past porno theaters and the prostitute hangouts. Finally we turned onto her street and stopped outside an apartment building on a beautiful old boulevard that had once been grand.

We went in. As we did Vicky turned and said, "I can't believe you're coming in here with me. Do you know who you are? You're Jill Ireland."

This made me uncomfortable and she repeated, "Do you know who you are?"

"No," I replied, "not at all."

Vicky unbolted the two locks on her door and we entered a small, dark room with a mottled orange-and-brown wool rug. It was full of boxes of papers, books, and clothes that hadn't yet been unpacked. The window was high and did not let in much light.

There was a couch against one wall and a single divan against the other. I did not want to look around in case she thought me critical. A long-haired tabby cat in good condition sprang to meet us. I picked him up and hugged him and made much of him. He began to purr.

"Look at the way he came to you," Vicky said. "I can tell about people by my cat. He doesn't like everybody. He likes you." She looked embarrassed, "Please don't judge me by this."

"Oh, Vicky, I'm not judgmental. I'm sure it's only temporary."

I remembered the photographs of her children, now in my purse so that I could show them to Charlie. They had been posed in front of Christmas trees at various ages in comfortable, homelike surroundings. This woman had done her best to rear three sons. She was a mother and a grandmother.

We sat together on the old leather couch. There was a copy of *Life Wish* on a pillow.

"It was a mistake, wasn't it, Vicky?" I asked. "You aren't the sort of woman to give up a child. It didn't suit you, did it?"

"No," she said. "But if I hadn't he would have had such a terrible life."

"Well, Vicky, I've kept him safe for you so far. And now we can share him."

She looked at me amazed and said she couldn't believe her ears.

"Would you really want to share him?" she said.

"Oh, yes. I would. You've no idea how wonderful it is and what a relief it is to meet someone who loves him as much as I do—that someone else can give him unconditional love. I've felt so alone with it all these years. Since I made contact with you, I've felt the pain of anguish ease. I'm able to understand for the first time that it might be possible for me to let go."

We spent a little more time together, then I told her I had to leave.

We hugged each other.

As I got into my car Vicky stood on the steps outside the building.

Her hands were clasped before her. She looked alone and my heart reached out to her, as it always did and always would reach out to her son.

I drove back through the dismal Hollywood streets, back along Sunset, retracing the last twenty-five years of my life, from Hollywood to Beverly Hills to Bel Air to Malibu. In spite of everything, I had been the lucky one. I had had those sweet baby arms around my neck. I had had the fingers entwined in my hair. It had been for me he had taken his first faltering steps. I had caught him as he fell, laughing with glee, into my arms.

I had had all that.

I felt so sorry for Vicky. She had lost one son whom she had loved with the same passion that I had for what was perhaps his twin soul, Jason. I knew I could do nothing to alter the situation. It would be wrong for me to encourage or discourage any further meetings between Vicky and Jason, who at this point felt he no longer needed to see her again. But I hoped for both their sakes that one day in the future the three of us would sit down together and share a meal, hold hands, and look lovingly into each other's face.

66
Farewell

1988

Before returning to England, my mother accompanied me to Washington, D.C., where I testified before the United States Senate Subcommittee on Health and Welfare, chaired by Senator Edward M. Kennedy. I addressed the subject of the inclusion of coverage by Medicare of mammograms for elderly women for early detection of breast cancer.

Mummy was delighted to see the government in action, and the trip broke up her long flight back to Eastbourne. We had left Daddy in the care of my brother and Dino, our houseman, back at the Serra house in Malibu. I saw my mother off on her Concorde flight to London and returned home, in my usual state of exhaustion after cross-country airplane trips and the jet lag involved.

At the beach house I was transported back some forty-eight years as I studied a photograph taken when I was a child. I stood with my head tilted to the left. My ears hurt and my head throbbed. I raised both hands to my forehead, trying to seize the pain and draw it out like strands of thread. I could not.

My father stood behind me, his hands heavy on my shoulders. We were having our photograph taken—the only one that I can recall. Certainly it was the only one still in existence of we two when I was a little girl.

I was coming down with measles and the daylight's glare hurt my eyes, so I wore a large pair of dark glasses. Daddy was all-powerful in those days. I was just a doll, a tiny three-year-old figure, small, vulnerable legs, soft arms, almost helpless. He picked me up and carried me home.

Now he sat, puzzled, on a white couch at the beach house. He was trying to comprehend what I was saying but, having lost eighty percent of his hearing, complicated by the sound of the surf, it undoubtedly baffled his deaf ears. He hadn't quite understood.

"Daddy," I said in stentorian tones, "you should have a nice bath before you get on the plane. You will feel fresher."

"Ha?" he said, tilting his head and frowning at me and John.

My brother was agreeing with me enthusiastically. In fact the idea of giving Daddy a bath was uppermost in his mind.

John had flown in from Canada to accompany my father back to England.

"Dad," said my brother, "you've got to have a bath. And I can give you a nice, fresh change of clothes."

It was so strange that John and I kept telling him how *nice* everything was going to be. The bath, the change of clothes. But looking at the old man, sitting solidly like a huge gray-cashmere avocado on the couch, it was obvious that the very idea of shedding all his garments and getting precariously into a bathtub for the purpose of merely freshening up was not high on his list of priorities for the day.

However, John and I agreed that it was imperative that Daddy go back to the Serra house and bathe just before they departed for the airport. We began introducing the thought at ten-thirty in the morning and, having planted the seed that early, we hoped to nurture the notion throughout the day until the old man would actually think it was his idea. But so far, he just hadn't got it.

I sat beside him and tried again. "Daddy, listen. A bath; you've got to have a bath."

He heard me.

"Oaah," he said in a growling tone. "N'aaow."

"Yes, Daddy. You'll feel so fresh."

"Clean socks, Dad," John put in.

My father was flanked by his son and daughter. It was a day the three of them spent together, a unique occasion. So Daddy, perhaps wanting to please us, and perhaps just to get it over with, began removing his clothes. First his shoes and then the offending socks.

"No, Daddy, no. Not right now." I tried to stop him, but it was too late. The move was in operation. My father was going to take a bath right now. John and I both sprang to our feet at the same time.

"God," John said. "I don't have his clean clothes here."

I started the water running in the bathtub, squirting in bubble bath, and exited the bathroom just as my father staggered in, followed by my brother holding shoes, socks, and his sweater. John was chattering to Daddy's unhearing ears. The motion had been passed, and no matter what, Jack Ireland was going to take a bath and right now.

I could not help grinning as I closed the door on the two men. I heard much splashing:

"There you go, then.

"Steady!"

I could picture my brother lowering Daddy's disabled body into the water. This was a difficult maneuver because Daddy would allow no one to touch his right arm.

Soon John emerged. "I'm going to have to rush to the other house to get him a change," he said. "I'll be as quick as I can."

"All right, but Daddy will have to stay in the bath until you return, because I can't get him out."

John rushed out, leaving me alone with my soaking father. I sat at the table and looked out at the ocean.

"Aaarooo," came from the bathroom.

I sprang to my feet and ran to the bathroom door, opening it a crack. There lying in the bath, pink, round and as innocent as a newborn babe, both hands clasped over his private parts, was my father, his white head with its back to me, his hair wispy and fluffy. From the angle at which I stood at the door, he really did look like a young child, not an old man at all. His skin still held a baby-pink firmness.

"I'm here, Daddy," I shrieked as loud as I could. "Don't worry. I'm going to stay until John gets back. I'll be here."

"Aor," he said. Okay.

I knew how vulnerable he felt in the tub. In fact, I had had to relieve the male nurse of his duties, a man who stayed in our employ for a mere three weeks. My father didn't like him and resented the idea of a nurse. One day the man left my father in his bath for a very long time. My father had let the water out and called for assistance. No one came. He lay there cold and wet much longer than he deemed necessary. The following day he lost his temper with the nurse and raised his fist. The man, young, strong, and almost six-feet tall, said, "Don't you dare hit me."

And although none of us is sure if that was Daddy's intention to start with, having been thus challenged, Jack hauled off and punched the man, ending their relationship for good and all.

I hoped John wouldn't be too long with Daddy's clothes. I returned to the chair in the sitting room when he called again. I went to the bathroom door.

"It's all right, Daddy. I'm still here."

"Aah ah," he said, reassured.

I noticed he had begun washing his hair with his one good hand. John returned with remarkable alacrity with socks, underwear, a colostomy bag, clean trousers and shirt. He entered the bathroom with the efficiency of a midwife, and I heard him getting Daddy out of the bathtub.

"Talcum powder," he called.

I ran to get a box of dusting powder, which my brother sprinkled on Daddy's shoulders. Then John brought Daddy out wrapped in one of Charlie's white terrycloth robes. Now my father was pleased, rosy, clean, shampooed. I combed his hair for him and helped with his sock and shoes. Then I made scrambled eggs and toast and we three Irelands sat at a table looking out on the briny and congratulating ourselves on a job well done.

I wished at the end of his days that I could have lifted my father from the bath and rolled him up in a big warm fluffy bath towel as he had done for me a mere forty-eight years earlier. I hoped he had enjoyed those forty-eight years.

Well, I consoled myself, he had certainly enjoyed his lunch. The day passed pleasantly and when I saw my brother and father off on their long journey to England, it was with the anxiety of the separation of a mother from her child when she leaves him for the first time in nursery school. I kissed Daddy good-bye.

"Take care of him, John," I said.

Daddy stoically did not give in to tears as Charlie hugged him good-bye, and I could see he was looking forward to the airplane trip back and the adventure it would be.

Good-bye, Daddy. Good-bye. Good-bye.

67

Afterword

I should be enjoying, for the first time in my life, a lighthearted freedom from most of the worries of parenting. Now I cannot see that happening. Maybe one never attains that Nirvana, the cherished freedom from constant concern—a state of mind I had hoped one day to reach.

The situation with my elderly parents is one I face constantly. My mother still lives in England, taking care of my handicapped father. Although she is a tough old lady and manages better than she should, it is a situation from which she has no escape. The strain is telling. The plight of my parents seldom leaves my mind.

My mother's fierce determination to keep her home and independence, her desire to keep going against all odds, my father's desperate wish to do the same, are inspiring and heartbreaking to watch—or rather to listen to. It is on the telephone that I try to monitor and help this family of mine. My gallant, stubborn, and resilient Mummy still lies about her age. She became indignant when, during a recent terrible blizzard that beset England, neighbors, constantly told by television to keep an eye on the elderly, knocked on her door to inquire about her well-being. Mother was furious. She does not see herself as elderly. Her wisdom and sense of humor attest to this. All the same, she needs the support of our telephone conversations as she stays one step ahead of stress and fatigue.

My parents occupy at least half the portion of my brain allocated to worry. The other fifty percent is give over to Jason.

Jason, my middle son, is an alcoholic and a drug addict. Only now, after more than four years of living with this knowledge, somehow the pain is not as devastating as it once was. I wonder if it is a matter of diminishing trauma and that in years further along, perhaps I will even become accustomed to the roller-coaster pattern that constantly threatens my son's chances for a happy, normal life.

Sometimes when the situation on the British home front flares simultaneously with a Jason crisis, I feel as if I will break and splinter into pieces.

Daddy and Jason. I am only just beginning to be aware of how unfair my concern for the two of them has been to my other children and my mother.

I tend to protect and nurture the weakest, the most troubled. But I do have other beautiful, talented, and loving children—and they also have a claim to my thoughts, concern, and time.

I have a most deserving mother who did not visit me for two years, "because I'd rather send Jack to you so I can rest and have the house to myself."

My joys have been as intense as my tragedies. But I am learning to acknowledge that I'm not omnipotent, that life would go on without me. My loved ones cannot be protected, guided, and controlled by me all their lives. Nor do they want to be. Indeed, many of them have struggled in the fist of my determination for years.

My father desperately fights to keep his dignity, at great

cost to my mother. It is a delicate balance loving them both, watching my mother and father struggle for their independence. They are right to live out their lives in their own home. So I will let go or at least behave as if I have.

I will let everyone live his or her life, stop worrying, stop wondering how they are. Okay. All right. It's done. I've done it. But why do I feel as if I'm waiting for the other shoe to drop?

I cannot help but ponder the fate of Daddy's little girl, the one in the secure folds of the fluffy bath towel all those years ago. Is her fate the destiny of every Daddy's Little Girl?

Eternal motherhood?

Just sixteen years after "Red, Red Robin," I became a mother.

I find myself now parent to my three sons and two daughters, and in many ways parent to my parents.

Am I fated to eternal motherhood?

Where, I wonder, do I fit in?

Who is mother to me?

Am I pondering the problem of all women of my generation, the historical, traditional destiny of womankind, I wonder. Or is it unique to the twentieth century? Thanks to the intervention of medical science people are living years longer. In my grandparents' time one rarely dealt with the question of elderly parents. Indeed, a woman was elderly herself at an age when today's woman is striving in her career and looking toward the future.

By prolonging the adolescence of our children and the longevity of our parents my generation finds itself caught like Peter Pan in Never-Never Land.

Making room for our own space in time is becoming increasingly difficult.

When is it our turn?

How do we fit into life as our future, past, and present tug at us desperately in different directions?

Where is our time for peace? Our time for us?

Maybe we are the true lost generation.

I always feel as if I know what's best for my aging parents and my robust offspring. And, on paper, I do.

But as I become older and wiser, I realize only one individual knows what is best. That someone is the person still traveling the journey of his or her life, and not an observer, no matter how loving or related.

My children are old enough to bear children, and yet I constantly worry for each and every one of them. My mother told me that this never will end. So I am caught up in a vortex of parental concern that continues forever and ever and ever, spiraling down through the generations where it will eventually be taken up by the youngest member to spin it off to spiral yet again.

(Hey, Nooch. Guess what? Shotgun's here!)

November 7, 1989

"No! No!" Charlie shouted. "God, no!"

We were in our Vermont home. It was nearly midnight when the telephone rang in the kitchen. Charlie answered. I was sitting on a couch in the breakfast room, or the *breezeway* as we call it. Next to me sat my sister-in-law Sandra Ireland and her daughter Courtenay.

Again we heard the cry of "No!" and a chair being pulled away from a table as Charlie sat down.

Also in the room with me was my nurse, Marie Krebbs, who told me much later that when she heard the chair scrape and Charlie's shock, she knew what had happened. But I suspected nothing.

I went into the kitchen.

What could have brought on such an outburst?

My first thought was news of a fire near our home in Malibu or perhaps one of the water pipes had burst there. I sensed the call had come from my eldest son Paul who was house-sitting for us. With some impatience and anxiety I entered the kitchen saying, "For heaven's sake, Charlie, what is it?"

My urgency after hearing his painful words was based in fear probably, but at that time I didn't know it.

He turned and looked at me.

"My God! Jason's dead."

Charlie looked to be in deep shock.

I sank into the nearest chair, a wooden ladderback, one of four around the kitchen table.

Sandra came into the room immediately, arms at the ready, to comfort me, followed by Marie. Courtenay burst into tears and ran upstairs to her bedroom.

I greeted the two women with cold eyes. I didn't want anyone's comfort. I did not cry. I just sat there, numb. I couldn't believe it. Jason, dead. I tried it on in my mind. It didn't feel true. Not right somehow. I turned my back on everyone and walked into the sitting room. I needed to be alone. I huddled in the big chair in the corner, the same chair that held me five years earlier when I learned of Jason's drug addiction, the day I had picked up the telephone extension and heard the fateful words, "The kid is on the needle."

Once again it was here in this house that I was absorbing more horror. The first time I had cried, sobbed, screamed, "No, Jason. No!" But not now. An icy coldness came over me. I wanted no relief from tears and no comfort from anyone.

I began making phone calls to people who knew him. "Jason's dead," I would say tersely.

"No! No!" was always the response.

"Yes," I would say harshly. "I'll call you back with more information. I'll be flying to Los Angeles tomorrow."

Charlie entered the room. "Jill, you can't go to L.A. You must stay here. I'll go."

"No way," I said. "I'm going. There's no way I'm going to sit here while my son is buried. I *have* to go."

"But this is the dangerous time," Charlie said desperately. "Your white blood cell count is down. You're too weak to make that trip. You can't expose yourself to all the people at the funeral. Jill, I'll be devastated if this destroys your health."

Charlie had good reason to worry. For eighteen months I had been fighting cancer again, first with extreme radiation treatment, chemotherapy and radiation implants.

Then I started a program of treatment. Every twenty-eight days I was admitted to Arlington Memorial Hospital in Texas. Under the direction of Dr. George Blumenschein, I received massive doses of chemotherapy. They were administered through a catheter implanted in my chest. Dr. Samuel Jampolis inserted the vital radiation implants. I also underwent three surgeries in a week before going to Vermont.

My life had been severely threatened by a quart and a half of liquid accumulated in the sac, called the pericardium, surrounding my heart. Another quart and a half of body fluid had accumulated in my lung. I had been walking around with 17½ pounds of liquid in my chest. Small wonder I had had difficulty breathing. Now I was recovering in Vermont. Yes, Charlie had reason to worry.

But I was full of a steely, angry determination. I was going home to bury Jason. Nothing would stop me.

That night, away from well-meaning eyes, I let go and cried. I was joined, shortly, by Charlie. We both grieved and cried for most of the night.

We are very private people. We keep our weeping for our private times.

The next day we flew to Los Angeles. Paul greeted us at our Malibu home. He was in charge, ready to take over all responsibilities. As usual, Paul was strong, reliable and I was proud.

"I love you, Paul," I said as we embraced.

"I love you, little mother," was his reply.

No tears were shed. My Englishman was strong for me. He knew it was important for me to preserve my strength, to ration it out through the next few days. There would be time enough for mourning after the funeral. Then many tears would be shed, for Jason was much beloved.

Next to greet me was David McCallum. We held each other and looked long into each other's faces. No tears here either, just an infinite sadness and understanding.

We entered the house together. Suddenly my daughter, my heart, was hugging me tightly. Her hugs are always so special, but this one, oh this one. . . .

Next came my lovable six-foot-six Englishman, my great galoofer, Valentine. "Hi, Mom," he said in a choked voice.

"Hi, sweetheart."

He bent down to hug me. I could see he was hurting terribly. It was in his eyes. But there were things to do, things to be decided. No tears shed yet. At least not together.

While Charlie and I fielded telephone calls, Paul made arrangements for the funeral. The night before the services, Charlie and I went to see Jason for the last time. Paul had chosen his clothes, so I knew Jason would be wearing a white shirt, dark blazer and black jeans. I had fought against an autopsy. I couldn't bear the thought of his poor body being cut, although reason told me he was at peace now and past pain. Yet somehow I still hated the thought of him being further violated. But I was told it was a legality, something that could not be avoided.

I had slipped into my purse a small pair of scissors and a rosary of white seed pearls a well-wisher had sent me. I am not a Roman Catholic, but this symbol of love had comforted me during my trials with my health for many months. I planned to leave it with Jason. The scissors were to cut his hair, a lock for me, a lock for Paul and a lock for Valentine.

Charlie and I entered the mortuary with its plush carpet and curious stillness. This was not a house of the living. As we entered the elevator, I felt the panic start. By the time we arrived at the third floor, I was shaking. The man who showed us the way opened the large polished oak door and ushered us into the room before leaving us alone.

I cannot describe the pain of seeing my child in his coffin. It was his face and yet it wasn't. They were his hands and yet they weren't. His hair, long and luxuriant, was definitely his hair. I took out a hairbrush and began brushing it, sobbing deep gasping sobs, talking to him all the while as Charlie stood off watching helplessly. I told Jason I loved him. I kept asking him why. The pain in my chest was excruciating. But I could not stop sobbing, Oh, My God, Jason. Oh, Jason!

Then I cut three pieces of hair and placed them in separate envelopes. I wanted to place the rosary in his hands. But his fingers were locked, cold and hard, so I slipped it into his breast coat pocket.

I buried my face in his hair. It was the only thing that still seemed to hold a part of Jason. Although I knew it wasn't Jason, just the house he had lived in, it was still my Jason's body. My heart broke to see him there like that, so vulnerable, so final. I was fiercely protective. No one else was going to touch him ever again.

I pulled up the white velvet blanket that was folded down over his knees and tucked it up beneath his face as I had so many times over the years. I closed the casket and asked Charlie to call the attendant to lock it. I didn't want it opened again. I had planned an open-casket viewing before the funeral the following day. Now, having seen him, I changed my plans. I knew he would not want anyone else to see him that way. I hoped everyone would remember him as he had been, not as he now looked. I had used an entire box of Kleenex. It was time to leave this room of grief. Charlie and I had said our goodbyes to the little boy and the young man whom we had had for such a short time.

Because of the extremity of my grief the previous evening, I was able to get through the funeral without breaking down. The services were dignified and quite beautiful. They began with a short and simple service by a Protestant pastor.

Paul gave a beautiful talk. He spoke of Jason as a little boy:

"I was lying on my bed with a terrible headache. The room was dark and I felt someone stroke my head gently, kiss me on the cheek, and say, 'You're going to be all right, Paul. Everything is going to be all right.' It was the sort of kindness that came from our mother in our family. This time it was the five-year-old Jason.

"That kid of love and giving is what Jason was all about. That was the kind of person our family knew.

"Everybody here has secrets and things about themselves they try to hide. One thing I admired about Jason was the strength he had to be himself and not hide the negative things about himself. Jason wasn't a hypocrite. He was very honest about what he was."

Paul said he and Valentine had reminisced about Jason the previous night, laughing at anecdotes, recalling the time as a child when Jason had eaten Paul's pet caterpillar.

"The best laughs in our family came from Jason, and that is what we'll miss the most," Paul said.

Next Valentine stood up with his guitar and said, "This was Jason's favorite piece. I wrote it some time ago.

"Jay-Jay, this is for you. I love you."

Then he was joined by Paul with his guitar and their close friend Charles Bishart on the violin. The trio played a hauntingly sad tune. Many people wept.

When my boys returned to their seats, Valentine, aware that it would be the last time he played that song for Jason, gave way to wracking sobs, his shoulders shaking with grief. Paul pressed Valentine's head to his chest and comforted his younger brother for several minutes until Val regained his composure.

I felt curiously weightless. I saw the mourners file past the casket to pay their last respects. I know I walked to the car and was driven to where the interment would take place. I saw the six pallbearers, Tony, Paul, Valentine, Cory Greenfield, David and Charlie, carry the coffin to the grave site.

I locked eyes with Katrina when the minister began reading a poem, the same one I had chosen for Katrina's mother's service and that was engraved on her plaque.

The chapel had been full of rather establishment-type people. The pews were full of Jason's friends, my friends and Charlie's friends, properly attired in business suits and neckties.

As the automobile procession formed and proceeded from the chapel to the grave site, I saw from the limousine window a young rocker on a motorcycle with long, dark hair almost to his waist, a red bandana over his head, a sleeveless leather vest, his arms decorated with an array of tattoos. He revved the motorcycle ahead of the procession in front of the hearse, rather like an honor guard.

I was relieved to see this bit of flamboyance. Even in my numb state, I felt that the urbanity of everyone's dress made it hard to believe this was Jason's funeral. Jason would have approved. I learned later the motorcyclist's name was Nadar, that he was a member of a group called London, and was planning to dedicate his next album to Jason.

We buried Jason in the same cemetery where Dempsey, Charlie's brother, was buried. Jason had loved Dempsey deeply and the idea of them being together pleased us all. But no one as much as Suzanne, who crossed the sixty feet or so to Dempsey's grave marker, and looking contemplatively she said, "Hey, Nooch. Guess what? Shotgun's here!"

A familiar greeting from Dempsey was "Hey, Nooch," no matter what other nickname the person had. What can I say, Dempsey was a nickname person. Shotgun had been Jason's nickname since childhood. But it took Suzanne to remember.

Next came a harsh moment. I found somebody's eyes burning into me and I turned to see Judy Brown, previously called Vicky in this book. But she has since identified herself to the press so I see no further need to protect her identity. I looked at her and smiled sympathetically and mouthed the words, "Hello, Judy."

She responded with a glare of pure hatred that went right through me. At this open, vulnerable moment, it hurt. I thought I had only been kind to Judy. I took the smile from my face and gave her one last look before turning my head away. With that turn of my head, I severed all connection with the woman who I had honored up to this moment out of respect for Jason.

I later learned that when I left the burial site, she posed for photographers flinging herself on the coffin and attempting to pry it open, all the while being photographed by the tabloids.

A few days later Judy called our business office saying she would like a sentimental little token, something to keep, that belonged to Jason. "How about his (Isuzu) truck," she suggested. But I had turned my head and whereas I once would gladly have given her the automobile, I had turned away from her forever.

My son was dead. There was no further reason to waste time or thoughts on Judy Brown.

Jason and I had spoken two days before his death. His last words were: "I love you, Mom. Don't worry about me. I don't want you to be stressed. I'm worried about you."

We reassured each other that we were fine.

"Don't worry, Jason."

"Don't worry, Mom."

He sounded optimistic and happy and I believed him. Now I knew he would not want his death to harm me physically. So I returned to Texas after the funeral to continue my treatment. While I was there, I was told the Los Angeles County Coroner's office reported that Jason had died as a result of an accumulation and mixture of drugs in his system, some of them prescribed by doctors.

In spite of all my torment and tragedy, at the point of this writing, the treatment seems to be working and I am getting stronger day by day.

On the other home front, Lo Lo continues marching on, enjoying life, relishing the moment, fighting like a demon when my mother puts him in a nursing home for once-a-month breaks. My mother? She's flourishing.

Jason wanted one thing at the end. He wanted very much to do anything in his power to stop other people from becoming hooked on drugs. In a television interview, which aired the night after his death, Jason had said, "Don't do it. Don't start."

He also said, "A drug addict doesn't want to hurt anybody. I never wanted to hurt anybody. I just needed the drugs to keep myself feeling normal. I never meant to hurt anybody."

I believe this. I love you, Jason.

(Jill Ireland Bronson, Arlington, Texas, 1989)